Troubleshooting Histology Stains

For Churchill Livingstone

Publisher: Gavin Smith
Project Controller: Sarah Lowe
Copy Editor: Julie Gorman
Text Design: Charles Simpson
Cover Design: Jeannette Jacobs
Index: Nina Boyd

Troubleshooting Histology Stains

Richard W. Horobin
Department of Biomedical Science, The University of Sheffield, Sheffield, UK

John D. Bancroft
Histopathology Department, Pathology Directorate, University Hospital, Queen's Medical Centre, Nottingham, UK

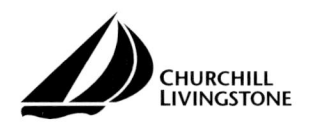

CHURCHILL LIVINGSTONE

NEW YORK EDINBURGH LONDON MADRID MELBOURNE SAN FRANCISCO AND TOKYO 1998

CHURCHILL LIVINGSTONE
Medical Division of Pearson Professional Limited

Distributed in the United States of America by Churchill Livingstone Inc., 650 Avenue of the Americas, New York, N.Y. 10011, and by associated companies, branches and representatives throughout the world.

© Pearson Professional Limited 1998

⬩ is a registered trademark of Pearson Professional Limited.

All rights reserved. No part of this publication may be reproduced, stored in a retrieval system, or transmitted in any form or by any means, electronic, mechanical, photocopying, recording or otherwise, without either the prior permission of the publishers (Churchill Livingstone, Robert Stevenson House, 1-3 Baxter's Place, Leith Walk, Edinburgh, EH1 3AF), or a licence permitting restricted copying in the United Kingdom issued by the Copyright Licensing Agency Ltd, 90 Tottenham Court Road, London, W1P 9HE.

ISBN   0 443 05312 X

British Library Cataloguing in Publication Data
A catalogue record for this book is available from the British Library.

Library of Congress Cataloging in Publication Data
A catalog record for this book is available from the Library of Congress.

Medical knowledge is constantly changing. As new information becomes available, changes in treatment, procedures, equipment and the use of drugs become necessary. The authors and the publishers have, as far as it is possible, taken care to ensure that the information given in the text is accurate and up to date. However, readers are strongly advised to confirm that the information, especially with regard to drug usage, complies with latest legislation and standards of practice.

The publisher's policy is to use **paper manufactured from sustainable forests**

Produced by Longman Asia Ltd, Hong Kong
CTPS/01

Contents

Preface ix

Introduction to the book and its use xi

Plate section

Individual Staining Procedures

1. Acid hematin for phospholipids 2
2. Alcian Blue: critical electrolyte concentration (CEC) method 6
3. Alcian Blue–periodic acid–Schiff (PAS) method for acid and neutral mucin 10
4. Aldehyde Fuchsin for elastic fibers and pancreatic β cells 14
5. Alizarin Red for calcium 18
6. Adenosine triphosphatase (ATPase) demonstration using calcium–cobalt for fiber typing 22
7. Azodye methods for acid phosphatase 26
8. Azodye methods for alkaline phosphatase: simultaneous coupling 32
9. Best's Carmine for glycogen 36
10. Chloroacetate esterase for mast and myeloid cells 40
11. Congo Red for amyloid (Highman's method) and related methods 44
12. Cresyl Fast Violet for nucleic acids in nervous tissue 48
13. Fast Green for basic proteins 52
14. Feulgen stain for DNA 56

15.	Fouchet technique for liver bile pigments	62
16.	Gimenez method for *Helicobacter pylori*	64
17.	Gomori's one-step trichrome	68
18.	Gordon and Sweet's stain for reticulin	72
19.	Gram stain for bacteria, including Gram–Twort and other variants	76
20.	Grimelius' silver method for argyrophil cells	82
21.	Grocott hexamine (methamine) silver for fungi	84
22.	Hematoxylin and Eosin as an oversight stain	88
23.	Jones's hexamine silver method for basement membranes and basal laminae	94
24.	Lactase by an indigogenic method	98
25.	Leucine aminopeptidase for demonstration of proteases	100
26.	Luxol Fast Blue for myelin	106
27.	Masson–Fontana procedure for melanin and other argentaffin materials	110
28.	Masson's Trichrome	114
29.	Methyl Green–Pyronin for plasma cells	118
30.	Miller's elastin stain: a modified Weigert technique	124
31.	MSB technique for fibrin and other acidophilic materials	128
32.	Myoadenylate deaminase for muscle-fiber typing	132
33.	NADH diaphorase for muscle biopsies	134
34.	Nonspecific esterase using an azodye method	138
35.	Nile Blue sulfate for neutral and acidic lipids	142
36.	Oil Red O for fats	146
37.	Papanicolaou stains for cytology	150
38.	The periodic acid–Schiff (PAS) procedure for polysaccharides	154
39.	Perls' Prussian Blue for ferric iron	160

40.	Phloxine–Tartrazine technique for viral inclusions	164
41.	Phosphorylase for muscle-fiber typing	168
42.	Phosphotungstic acid hematoxylin (PTAH)	172
43.	Romanowsky–Giemsa stains	176
44.	Rubeanic acid method for copper	182
45.	Shikata Orcein method for hepatitis B antigen	186
46.	Solochrome Cyanine for myelin staining	190
47.	Southgate's Mucicarmine stain for mucins	194
48.	Succinate dehydrogenase demonstration by an azodye method	198
49.	Sucrase, by an azodye method	202
50.	Sudan Black for lipids	206
51.	Thiocholine cholinesterase method	210
52.	Thioflavine T method for amyloid	214
53.	Toluidine Blue for basophilia and metachromasia, and as an oversight stain	218
54.	Van Gieson's and other picrotrichrome oversight and collagen stains	222
55.	Von Kossa technique for mineralized bone	228
56.	Warthin–Starry method for spirochetes	232
57.	Ziehl–Neelsen and related stains of acid-fast bacteria	236
58.	Ziehl–Neelsen technique modified for leprosy bacilli	242

References	247
Where to find technical details of staining methods	257
Index	263

Preface

For much of our working lives we have been fascinated by how microscopic stains work. Our interest has always been of a practical nature, so, as well as working and researching in this field, we have helped teach scientific/technical staff in higher education institutions, and run professional training courses with groups such as the Royal Microscopical Society. Over the same time period our interests included a related issue: how to troubleshoot routine staining procedures.

Originally, one of us (R.W.H.) was particularly concerned with effects of impurities in commercial stains on staining performance; and still is involved, currently being a member of the USA Biological Stain Commission. More recently, however, our troubleshooting efforts have broadened in scope, to include topics such as microwaving in histopathology, and staining specimens embedded in water-miscible resins. A particular focus is the communications aspect of troubleshooting. How can experienced workers pass along their wisdom to beginners? This is increasingly important as the pace of methodological change accelerates, and we are expected to be familiar with a widening range of procedures. This book grew out of this context, reflecting our concerns.

Consequently, this book represents an interaction of two elements. Namely, a hard scientific background, plus a determination to address the day-to-day issues of the technologist at the bench. So, in the hope that this book can be made even better in future editions, we invite you to write to us with your experiences of using it.

Sheffield, UK Richard W. Horobin
Nottingham, UK John D. Bancroft

Introduction to the book and its use

Who was this book written for?

The authors had the practical benchworker in mind when writing this book. In particular, someone using a method for the first time, whether a novice in the field, or a person inexperienced with some particular procedure. So how will this book help you? It is not a staining manual, but a source of suggestions for avoiding staining problems. Or, if that strategy fails, for solving the problems. Read this book before carrying out a method which is new to you. Read it if something goes wrong. Read it if your local expert is not available, since the advice given is largely obtained from such experts.

What is the scope of the book?

With a few exceptions, the book considers procedures the staining reagents of which are dyes or their derivatives. Within these limits the routine and special stains of the cytologist, histopathologist and hematologist are addressed. Therefore immunostaining, in vitro hybridization and so on are not discussed, although a number of frequently used enzyme histochemical stains used diagnostically are considered.

The book deals with problems due to the staining processes, as well as those due to staining reagents. For instance, the effects of staining temperature and timing are considered, as well as the consequences of using impure dyes or unstable staining reagents. There is no claim made for encyclopedic coverage, either of procedures or of variants. If your favorite procedure is missing, write to the authors!

What kind of help will you find here?

The book is built around a core of individual entries, each dealing with a staining method and its variants. Each entry includes several kinds of information, always given in the following sequence.

Background material provides a context for subsequent sections. The chemical nature of the staining reagent is discussed here, as are the staining mechanism and common variants of the method.

Avoiding problems is the next topic. Comments are offered on ease of use, with the consequences of various embedding regimes being noted. After all, if you lack necessary skills or suitable reagents the best way of avoiding a problem may be to look for a different staining method. Finding suitable staining reagents, and ensuring that solutions remain effective, are also considered here, as are control procedures.

Identifying and troubleshooting problems are the next topics. The accounts parallel the ways in which problems come to the attention of benchworkers. Perhaps something is wrong with the staining reagent or staining solution? Is it the wrong color, or won't it dissolve? Or does the expected staining fail to occur? Or occurs only weakly? Or is staining of an unexpected color? Or does staining of unexpected structures take place?

Finally, suggestions for further reading are offered. These concern troubleshooting or understanding a procedure, or its potentially troublesome aspects. Books and articles cited here and elsewhere are listed at the back of the book.

Some points of nomenclature

A solution used for staining is termed a working solution. A dye must be made up at some particular concentration, and usually at some specific pH and so on, to constitute a working solution. This solution is sometimes produced just prior to use by mixing a buffer, or other solvent or solution, with a dye-containing stock solution. The stock solutions thus contain dyes at higher concentrations than the working solutions. Consequently, stock solutions need to be more stable than working solutions, to permit storage for longer periods of time. For this reason some contain additives, e.g. Romanowsky stock solutions contain organic solvents such as glycerol and methanol to prevent precipitation.

The nomenclature of dyestuffs is confusing. Most dyes were originally produced for industrial use, and such materials were given different tradenames by different manufacturers. Consequently, what one supplier offers as Basic Fuchsin, another may sell as Pararosanilin. Moreover, the numbers and letters attached to many dyes may vary, as does their significance. Pyronin Y and Pyronin G are, hopefully, the same dye. However, Alcian Blue 8G and Alcian Blue 5G are chemically different.

One way of reducing this confusion is to use the Colour Index (CI) nomenclature. This scheme allocates a unique description of either a CI number or name, or both, to each structurally distinct dye. Pyronin Y and G are both CI 45005. Alcian Blue 8G is CI Ingrain Blue 1, whereas Alcian Blue 5G is CI Ingrain Blue 8. Such descriptions are widely used in the standard handbooks (*Conn's Biological Stains* and the *Sigma–Aldrich Handbook of Stains, Dyes and Indicators*), and by many vendors of dyes. Some scientific authors use them, some do not.

Where did the information in this book come from?

Some information came from staining manuals, which typically contain relevant information under such headings as 'preparation of reagents', 'notes' or 'controls'. It did surprise us how little overlap there sometimes is in this respect between the different manuals. Another source of expertise was research papers, some of which are cited in this book. Other information was from the authors' laboratories, and the laboratories of their friends and colleagues. Indeed, conversations with experienced workers from other laboratories are a valuable, and underrated, source of knowledge. So if you, the reader, have information to add or criticisms to offer, do by all means write to the authors.

GENERIC ASPECTS OF AVOIDING OR SOLVING STAINING PROBLEMS

This book considers the standard stains used in light microscopy in biomedical settings, plus the more widely used special stains of the histopathology laboratory. The 'one stain at a time' format emphasizes artifacts and problems peculiar to individual methods.

Consequently, generic problems of specimen preparation, microtomy and specimen manipulation are underplayed. It is not possible to rectify this imbalance without writing another book, or indeed several more! However, in this preliminary section a few pointers are offered as an indication of how such generic problems can be avoided or dealt with.

DIFFICULTIES EXPERIENCED DURING MICROTOMY

1. The tissue block is too hard to cut. This can arise from overheating during infiltration.
2. The center of the tissue block crumbles on being cut. This may be due to poor infiltration by the embedding medium, which itself has many possible causes, from inadequate dehydration to insufficient impregnation time.

Damage to the tissue section visible to the naked eye

1. Sections are folded or creased. This can occur as sections are dried down onto slides. Folds can sometimes be avoided by careful handling, although some types of specimen fold very readily indeed.
2. Score marks and scratches cross the section. If these occur on all sections, a damaged knife blade is highly likely.

Damage to the tissue section seen down the microscope

1. 'Shattered' morphology occurs, limited to the center of a specimen. This has various possible causes, e.g. lack of penetration of fixative due to insufficient time in the fixative agent.
2. Hairline cracks run across the section. This can occur because of overchilling of the block face prior to cutting.

Staining artifacts

1. Staining of the slide surrounding the tissue is seen following hematoxylin and Eosin staining of paraffin sec-

tions. Application of excess protein-based adhesive is one cause of this.

2. The edges of the specimen are intensely stained, whilst the center is satisfactory. This can arise from various misadventures, e.g. overheating of the specimen during infiltration can 'cook' the outer layer of the specimen.

Contamination of tissue sections

1. Alien materials may be deposited onto the surface of sections. Such materials range from dust, to hairs and squames from the benchworker's skin, or even opportunistic fungi.

2. Fragments of adjacent sections may be deposited onto a section during floating out.

Artifacts of mounting and other poststaining manipulations

1. Refractile, or seemingly black, cell nuclei are seen in stained sections. This can occur if the dehydration following staining is incomplete, or if adequate de-waxing was not carried out.

2. Bubbles may surround the tissue if insufficient mounting medium was applied.

Plate section

Plate 1 Alcian Blue/PAS for mucins (see also Alcian Blue)

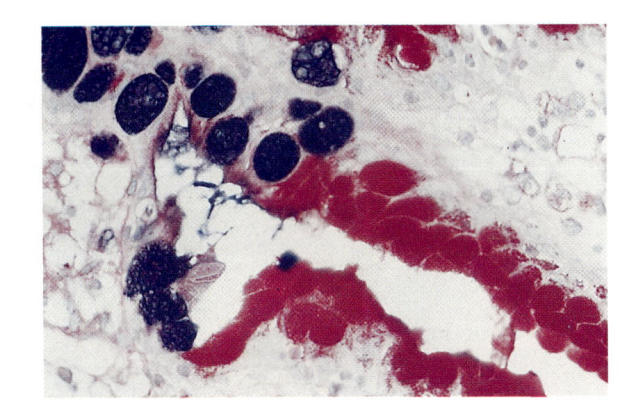

Plate 2 Aldehyde Fuchsin for elastin and ß cells

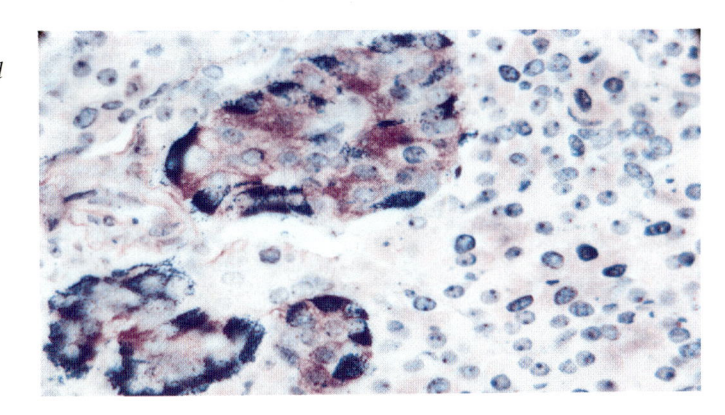

Plate 3 ATPase for fiber typing

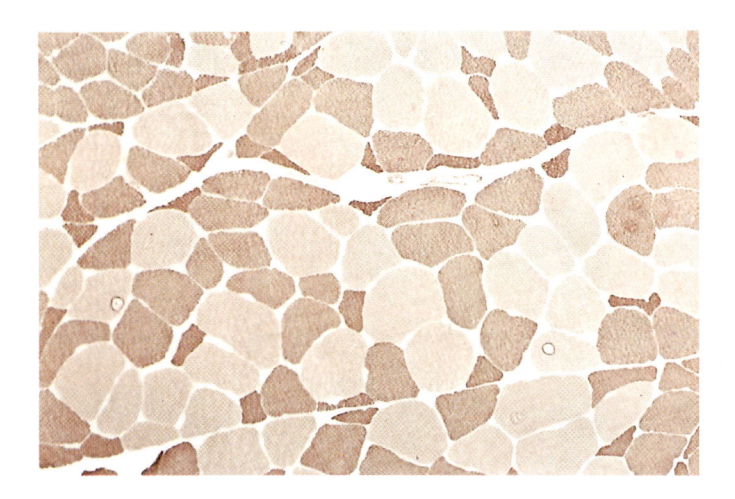

Plate section

Plate 4 Azodye methods for acid phosphatase

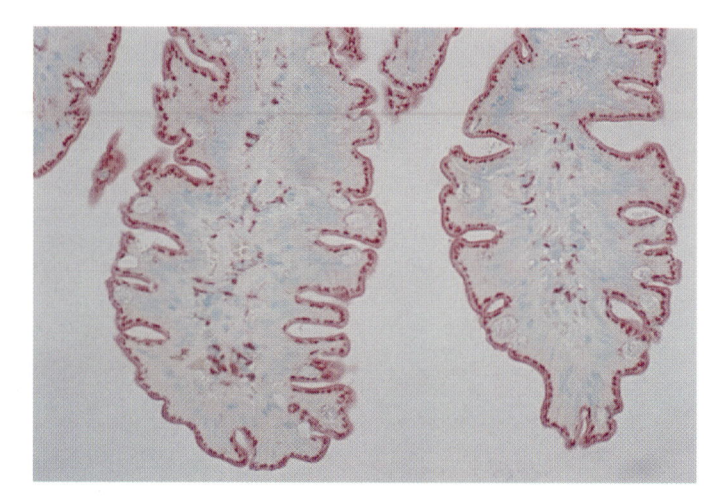

Plate 5 Chloroacetate esterase for myeloid and mast cells

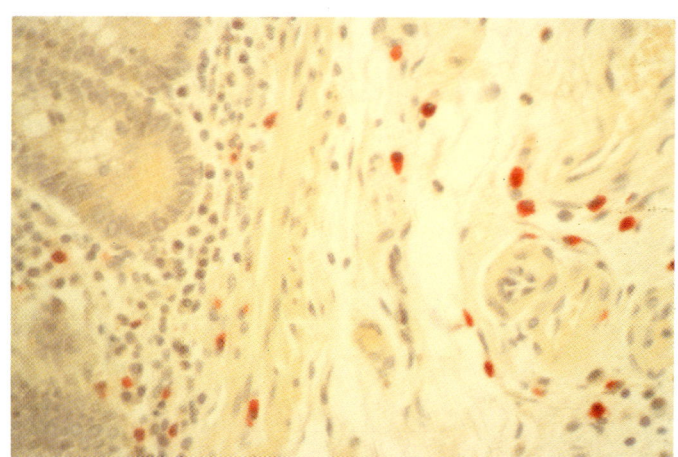

Plate 6 Congo Red for amyloid (Highman's method)

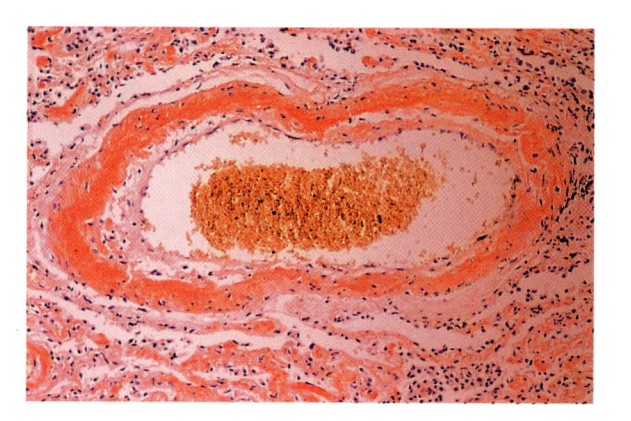

Plate section

Plate 7 Feulgen stain for DNA

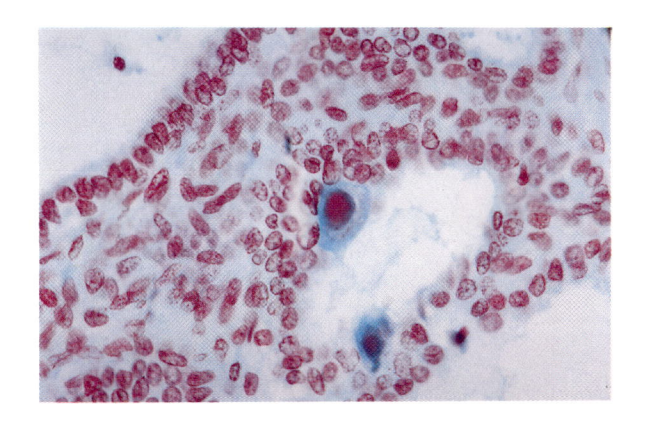

Plate 8 Fouchet for liver bile pigments

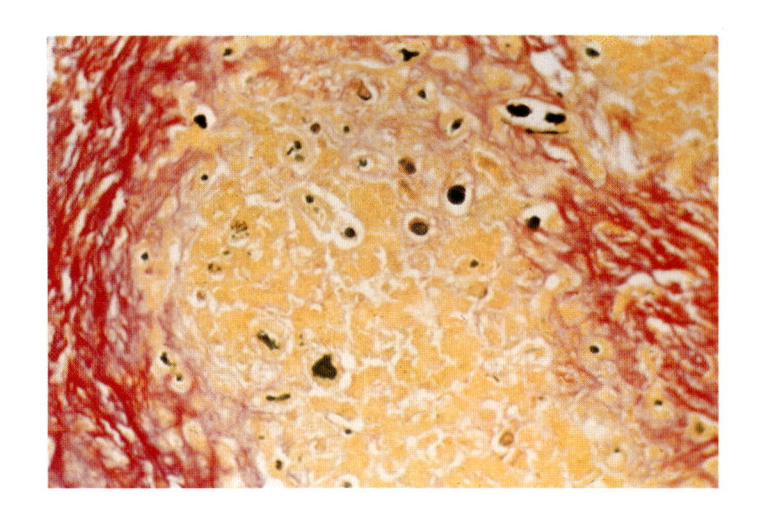

Plate 9 Gomori's one-step trichrome

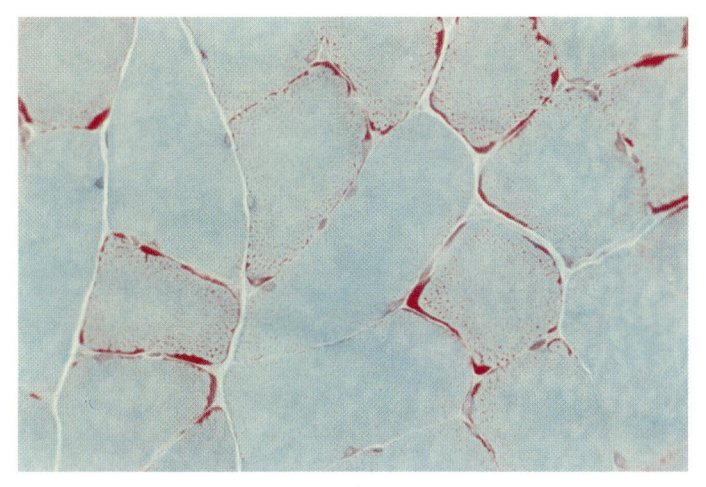

Plate section

Plate 10 Gordon and Sweet's stain for reticulin

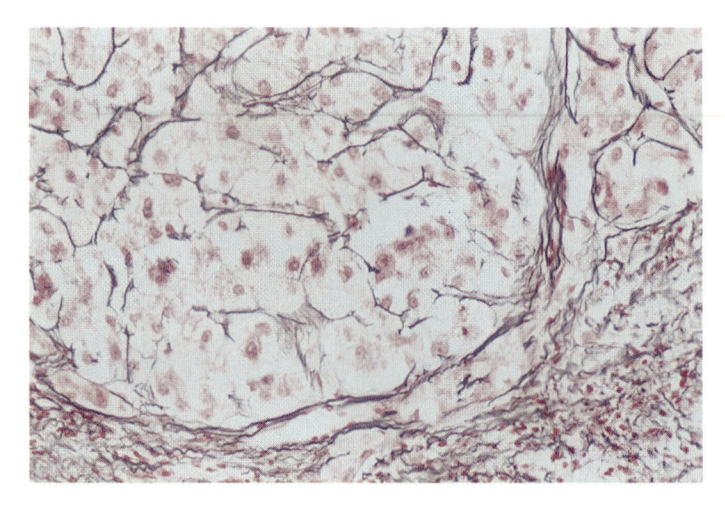

Plate 11 Gram stain for bacteria

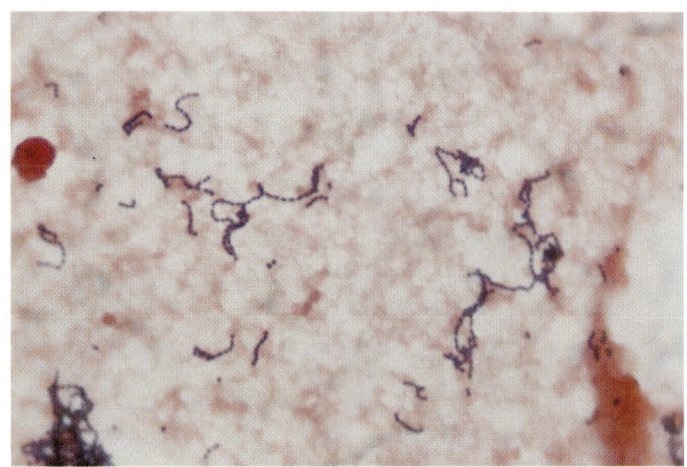

Plate 12 Grimelius' silver for argyrophil cells

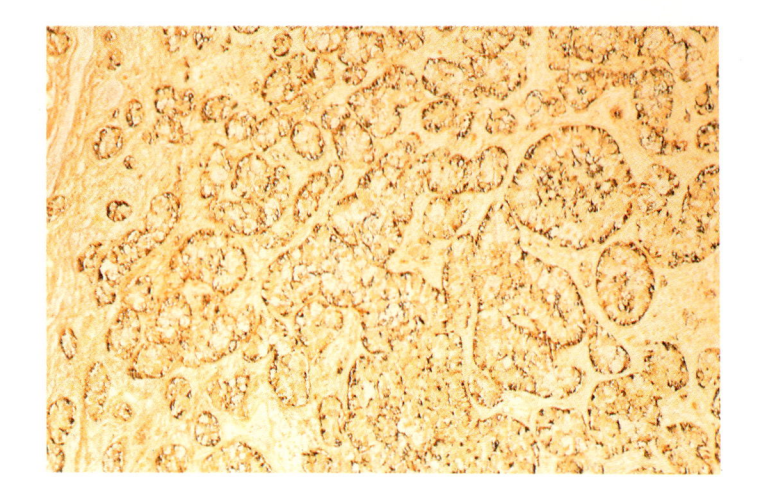

Plate section

Plate 13 Groccott hexamine silver for fungi

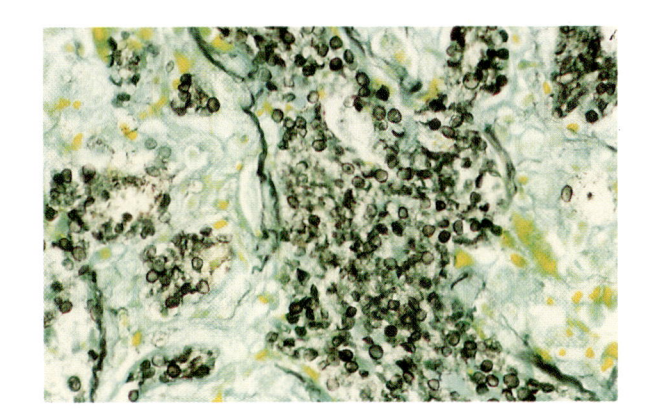

Plate 14 Jones's hexamine silver for basement membranes

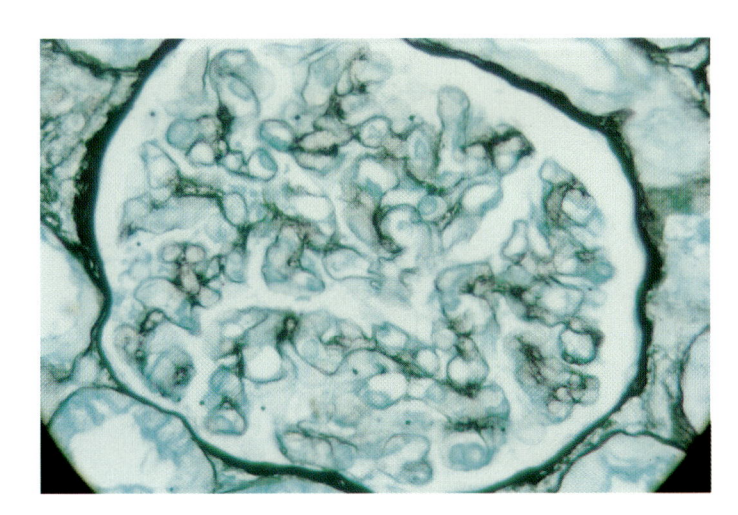

Plate 15 Leucine aminopeptidase demonstration

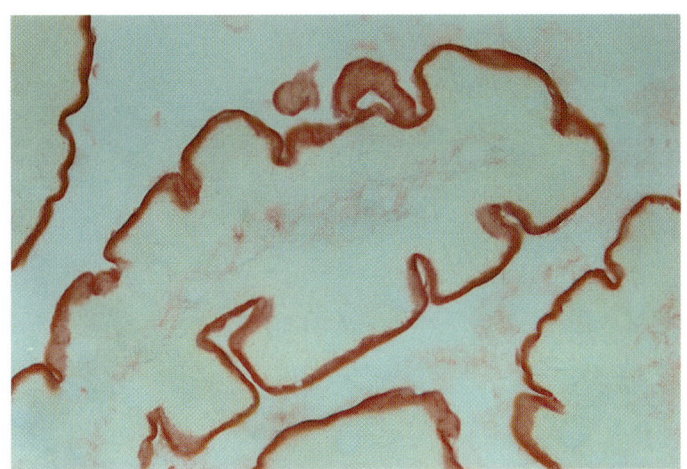

Plate section

Plate 16 Masson–Fontana method for melanin and argentaffin materials

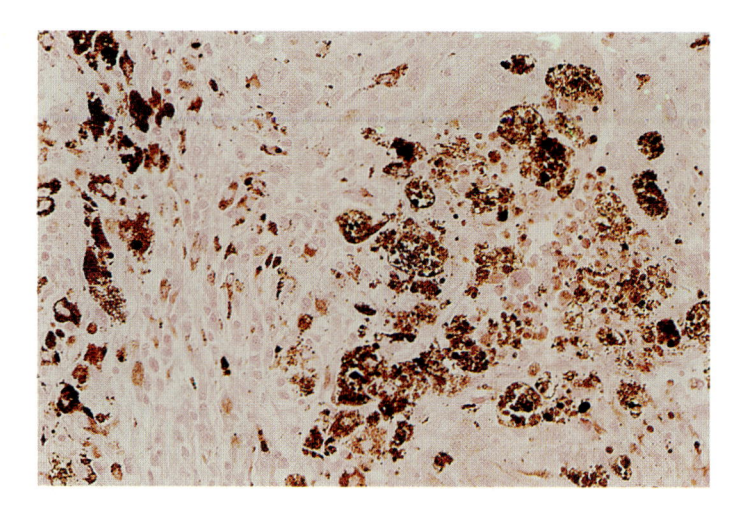

Plate 17 Methyl Green–pyronin for plasma cells

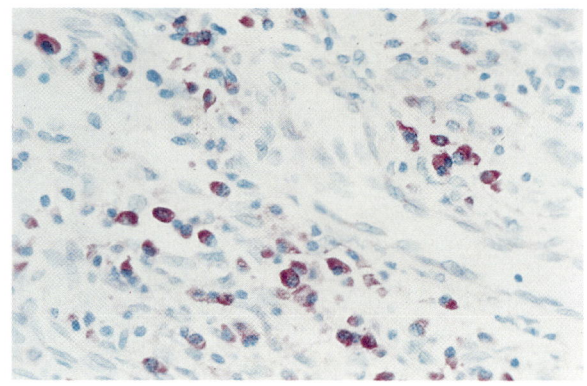

Plate 18 Miller's elastin stain

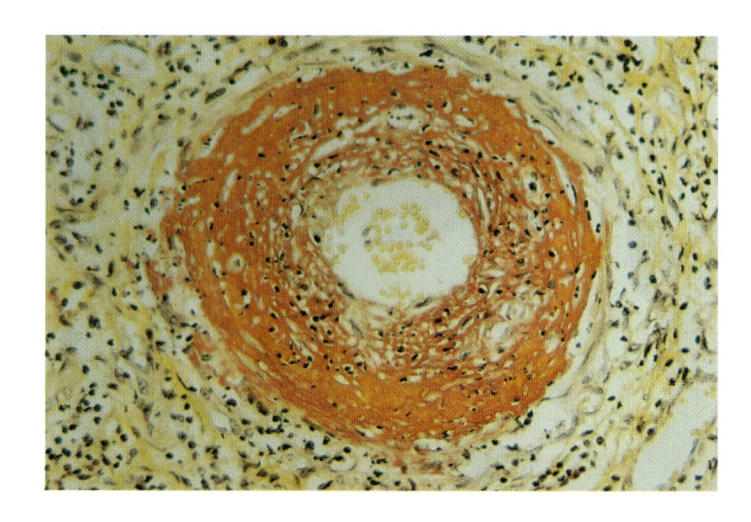

Plate section

Plate 19 MSB for fibrin

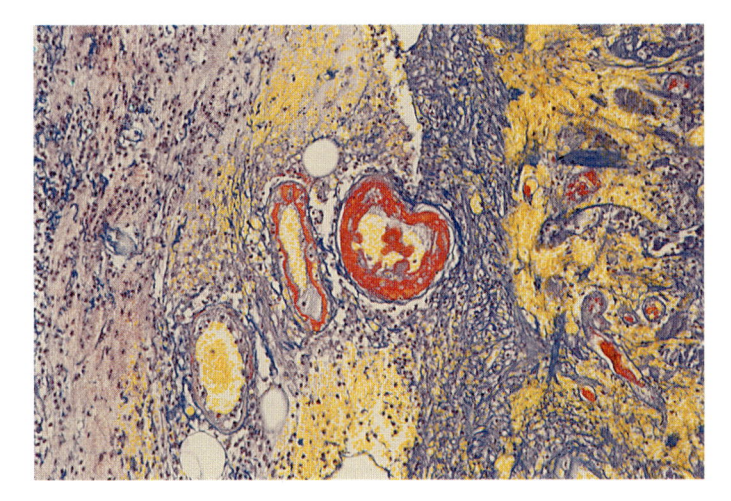

Plate 20 Nonspecific esterase azodye method

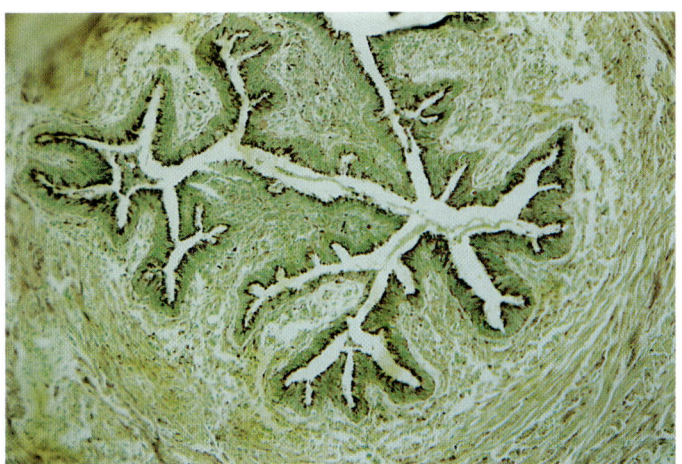

Plate 21 Oil Red O for fats

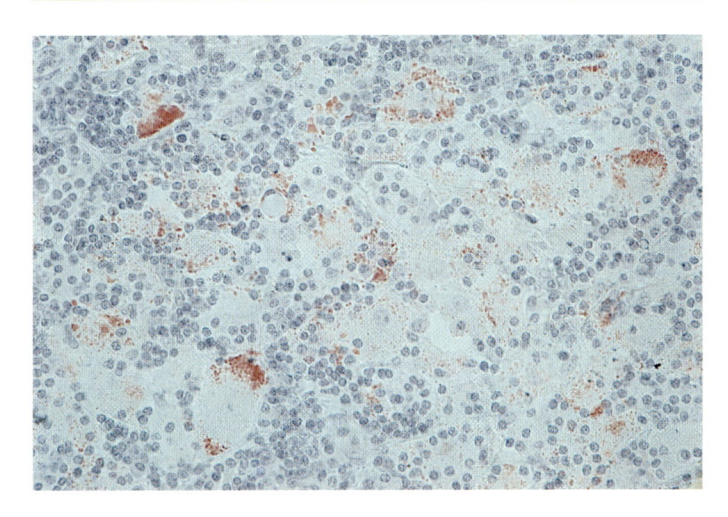

Plate section

Plate 22 Papanicolaou stains for cytology

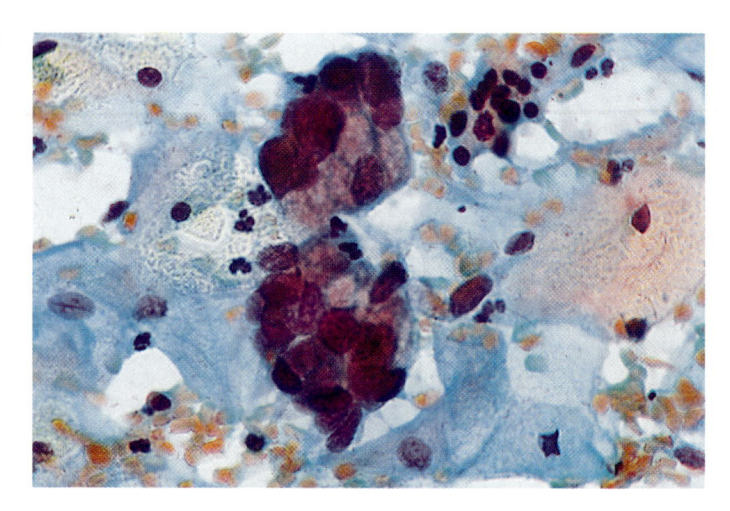

Plate 23 PAS for polysaccharides

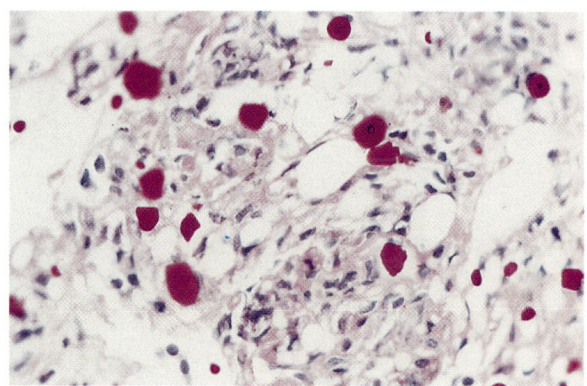

Plate 24 Perls' Prussian Blue for ferric iron

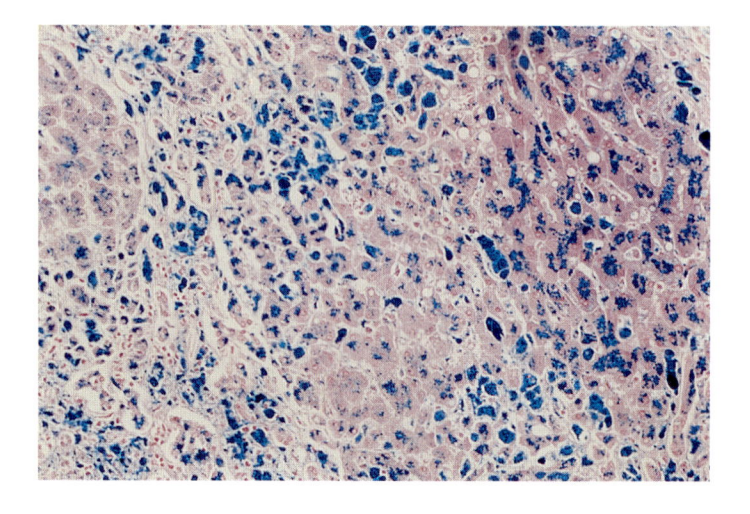

Plate section

*Plate 25
Phloxine–Tartrazine
for viral inclusions*

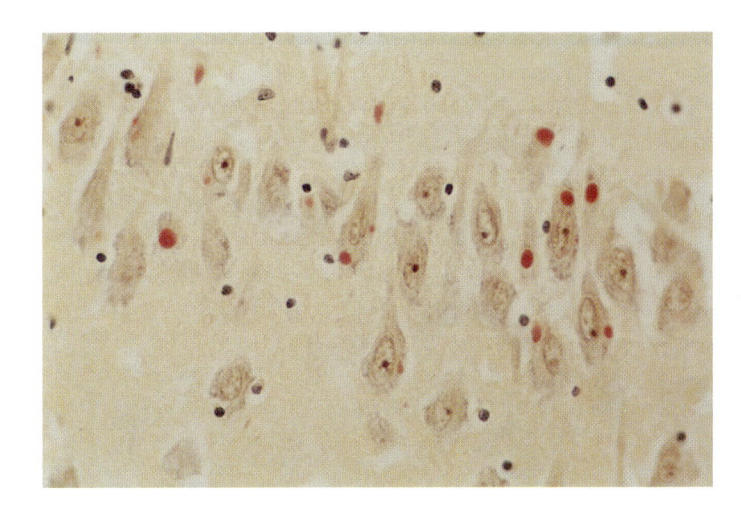

*Plate 26
Phosphorylase for
muscle fiber typing*

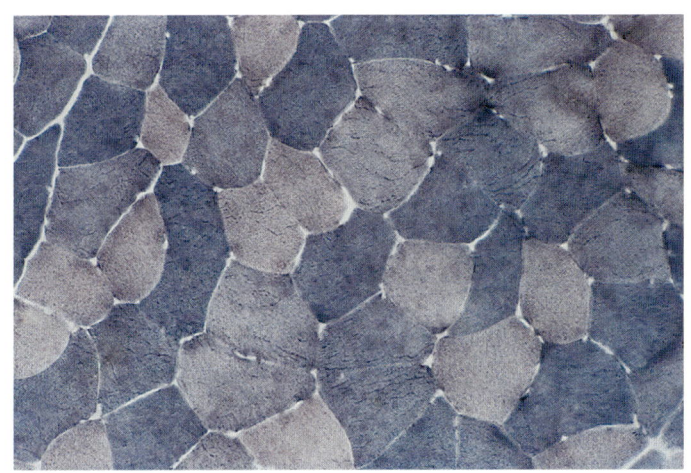

*Plate 27
Phosphotungstic acid
hematoxylin (PTAH)*

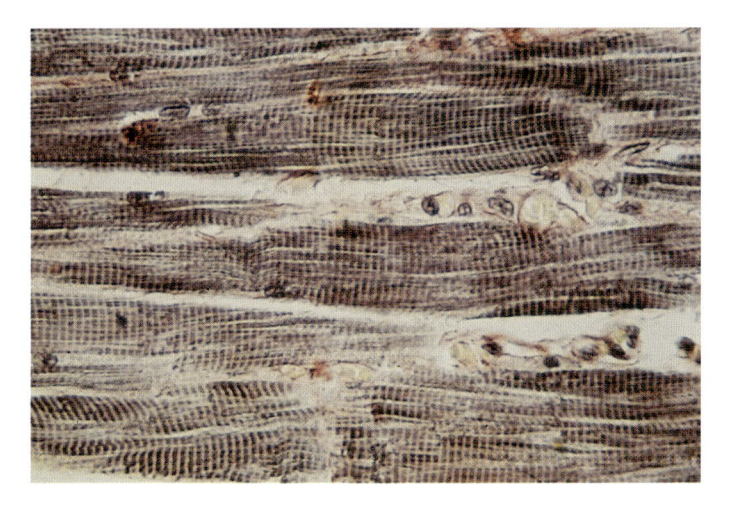

Plate 28
Romanowsky–Giemsa
stains

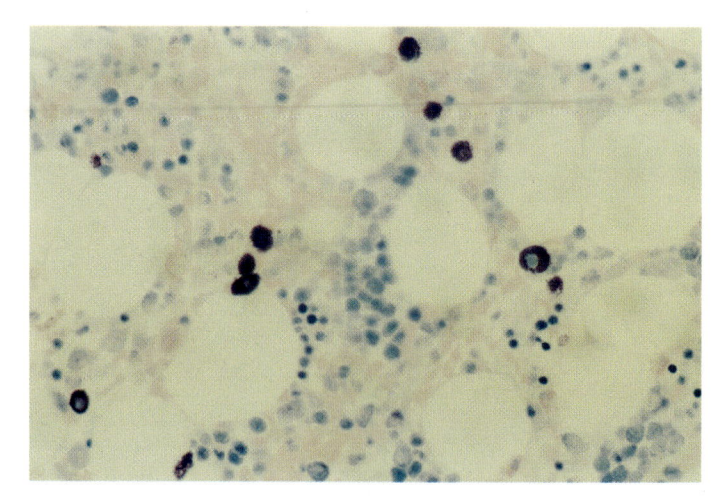

Plate 29 Rubeanic
acid for copper

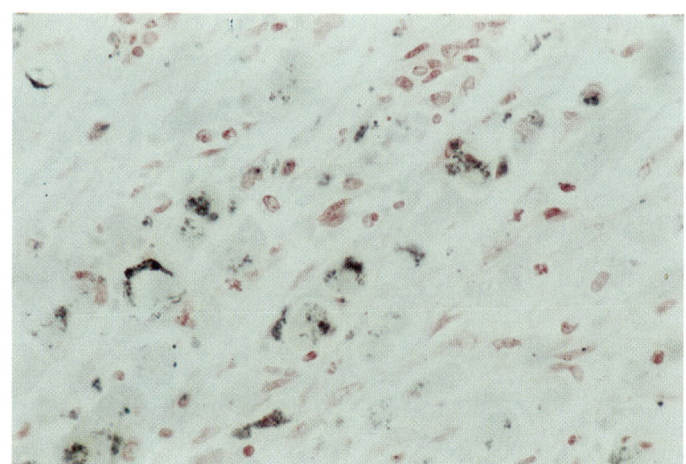

Plate 30 Shikata
Orcein for hepatitis B
antigen

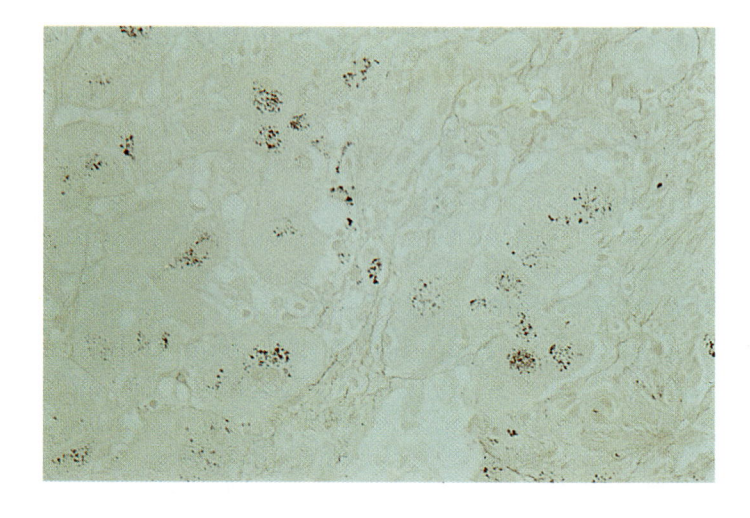

Plate section

Plate 31 Succinate dehydrogenase azodye method

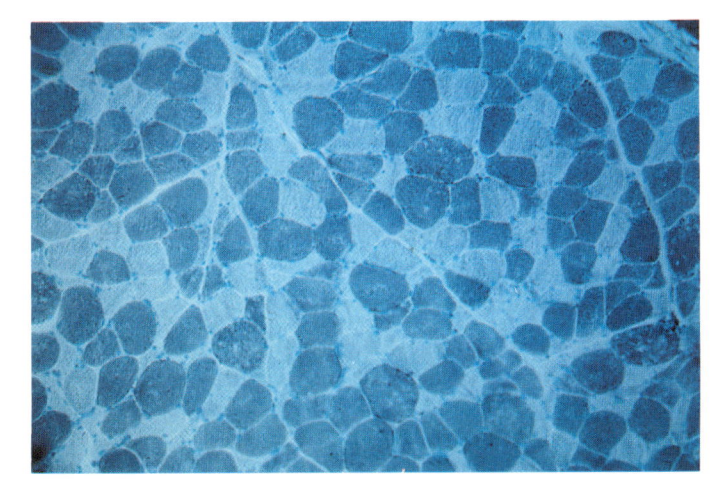

Plate 32 Toluidine Blue for basophilia and metachromasia

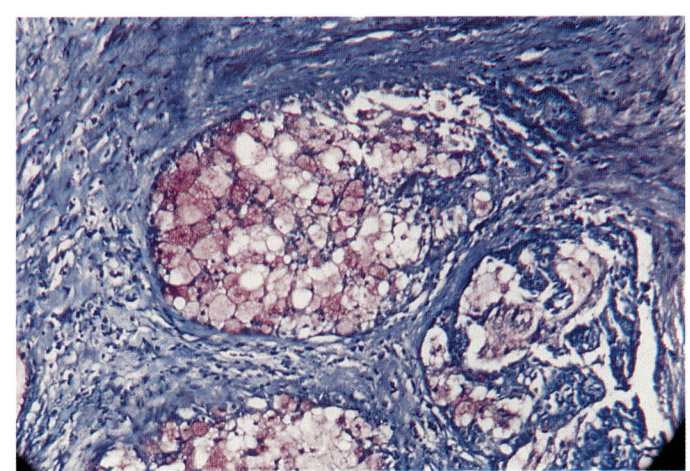

Plate 33 Von Kossa for mineralized bone

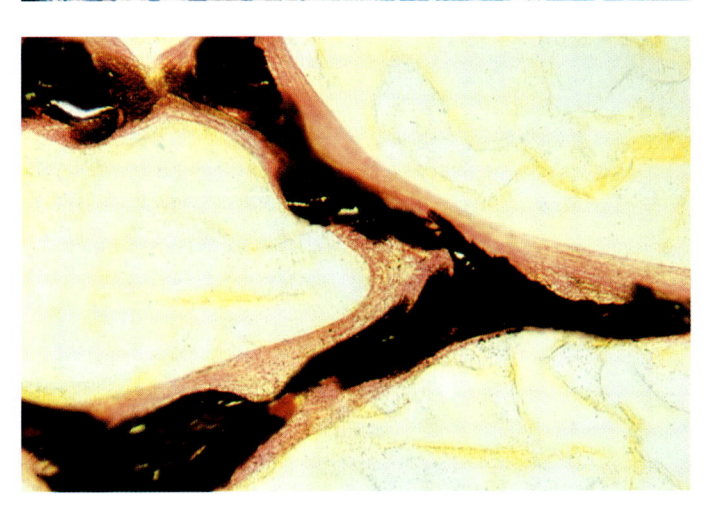

Plate section

*Plate 34
Warthin–Starry for spirochetes*

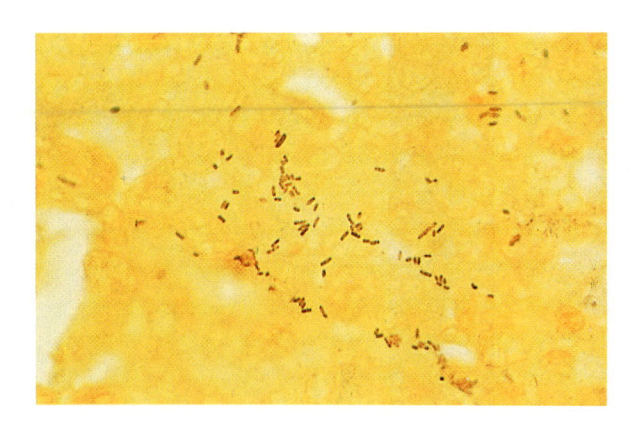

*Plate 35
Ziehl–Neelsen for acid-fast bacteria*

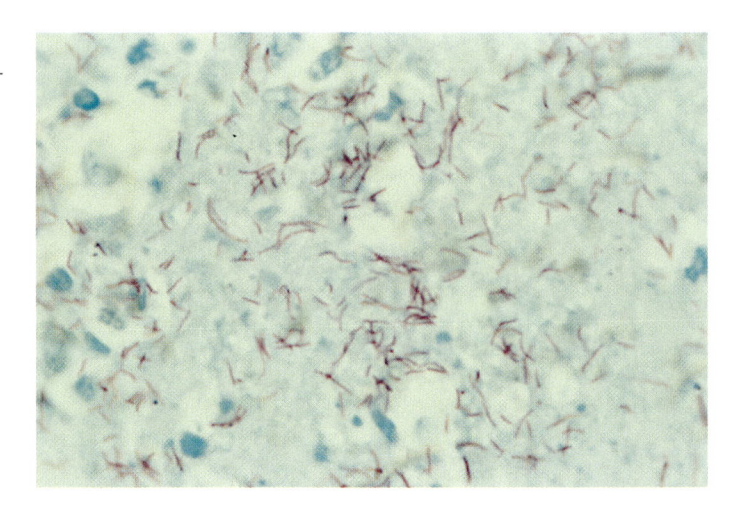

*Plate 36
Ziehl–Neelsen modified for leprosy bacilli*

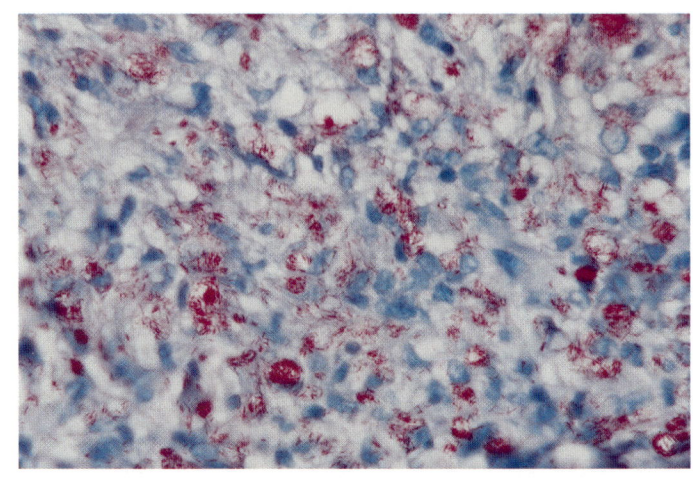

Individual Staining Procedures

1 Acid hematin for phospholipids

Background information

Hematoxylin is readily oxidized to form hematin, a lipophilic weak acid. This forms coordination complexes with a variety of metal ions, including chromium.

Specimens stained by acid hematin are first subjected to chromation, using potassium dichromate. This fixes lipids and attaches chromium ions to certain lipid-rich structures. The metal ions are visualized by an acidic hematin treatment. Background staining occurs, and differentiation in aqueous alkali is used to obtain selective staining.

Work using model systems suggested that dichromate reacts with, and chromium binds to, unsaturated fatty acids of certain phospholipids. Such chromium can be visualized by formation of colored coordination complexes with hematin (Chayen 1968). In tissues, however, dichromate will react with various substances, including proteins; the reduced chromium ions subsequently binding to a variety of ligands, including proteins (Hartley 1969, Elleder & Lojda 1970). Moreover, selectivity depends critically on subsequent differentiation, even in model systems (e.g. Roozemond 1971).

In tissue sections this will be more significant; and dense, protein-rich structures usually retain stain after differentiation, whilst diffuse, protein-rich structures do not. From this latter perspective, difficulties experienced when attempting to inhibit staining by prior lipid extraction are not surprising. However, such failures have been regarded by some as due to unmasking of phospholipids (Chayen & Bitensky 1991: 119).

Common variants

Essentially the same procedure is used under other names, e.g. Baker's acid hematin or dichromate–acid hematin. They differ with regard to chromation time or temperature, and time of the hematin treatment. However, the significant technical variable is probably the length of the differentiation time.

AVOIDING PROBLEMS

➤ **What types of specimen processing are suitable?**

Unfixed cryostat sections are preferred, or short-fixed frozen sections.

➤ **Is this procedure easy to carry out?**

With paraffin sections the method is manipulatively straightforward, although rather slow. However, despite reassurances from experts (Chayen & Bitensky 1991), the method is innately tricky. Selectivity is critically dependent on differentiation, and the solvent extraction control is itself of disputed validity.

Staining materials embedded in hydrophilic resins could prove difficult, since the acidic staining solution would tend to swell the resin, threatening section loss; and hematin, being hydrophobic, will itself stain the resin (see Horobin et al 1991).

➤ **Obtaining and keeping reliable reagents**

1. Use pure hematoxylin samples to prepare the acid hematin, not a difficult requirement as most commercial samples are of high quality.

2. Use the acid hematin on the day of preparation, since it is not stable.

➤ Useful routine control procedures

1. Carry out the staining method on a de-lipidized section, e.g. after immersion of sections for 1 h in acidic chloroform–methanol. The staining now seen will not be due to phospholipids. But note the opinions of Chayen (e.g. Chayen & Bitensky 1991: 119).

PROBLEMS AND HOW TO DEAL WITH THEM

➤ Tissue stains unexpectedly weakly

1. If stain is lost after dehydration or mounting, check that air drying or butanol dehydration, and an aqueous mountant, were used.

➤ Unexpected structures stain

1. Blue background staining may be due to retention of dichromate following chromation. Try extending the postchromation washing, to 24 h if necessary, or extending the borax differentiation time.

2. If stained structures are dense and protein-rich, suspect possible false-positives. Try staining a de-lipidized section whilst noting the ambiguities of such controls; or try differentiating for a longer period or at a higher temperature.

➤ Staining is of an unexpected color

1. On occasion some structures may stain deep brown, rather than shades of blue or black. Treat as valid positive staining on the basis of model system studies.

2. Occurrence of yellowish background staining is artifactual, probably due to reaction of hematin with tissue proteins, so ignore this.

Background reading

An optimistic account of the acid hematin procedure, and some discussion of its staining mechanisms is provided by Chayen (1968). More critical opinions, with yet more mechanistic arguments, can be found in Elleder & Lojda (1970) and Roozemond (1971). For relevant work on chromation from the textile dying context, see Hartley (1969).

2 Alcian Blue: critical electrolyte concentration (CEC) method

Background information

The dye required for the critical electrolyte concentration method is Alcian Blue 8G, whose major colored constituent carries four cationic substituents. Alcian Blue 5G and 7G are similar, but carry fewer of the cationic substituents and so are less water soluble. Alcian Blue 8GS and 8GX contain the same dye, but 8GX (X for extra) has a higher dye content than does 8GS (S for standard). After all this, note that in this entry, for 'Alcian Blue' read 'Alcian Blue 8G'.

Alcian Blue is a large, hydrophilic cationic dye. Its substantial planar phthalocyanine chromophore gives rise to marked aggregation in solution. Its isothiouronium groupings are chemically unstable. Thus exposure to hydroxide ion, or indeed to the nucleophilic groups that are plentiful in fixed tissue, result in formation of insoluble phthalocyanine pigments.

In the critical electrolyte concentration method, serial sections are exposed to slightly acidic Alcian Blue solutions containing varying concentrations of magnesium chloride. In high salt content dye-baths, staining intensities tend to fall.

Binding of Alcian Blue by anionic glycosaminoglycans is promoted by van der Waals attractions between Alcian Blue and tissue components, with selectivity for tissue anions being due to the cationic charge on the dye. The effects of the added salt are complex.

The originators of the procedure suggest that, under equilibrium conditions, dye cations and inorganic cations compete for tissue anions. Staining of carboxylated biopolymers is inhibited even at low salt concentrations, whereas sulfated biopolymers continue staining until higher salt concentrations. However, other mechanistic possibilities have been proposed, and several effects probably influence the staining patterns.

AVOIDING PROBLEMS

➤ What types of specimen processing are suitable?

The procedure can be applied to paraffin and cryosections, with mode of fixation not having been reported as of importance. For structures such as cartilage matrix or goblet cell mucin, this Alcian Blue method can be applied to tissue embedded in water-miscible resins such as glycolmethacrylate.

➤ Is this procedure easy to carry out?

The method is straightforward, the only common technical problem being poor solubility of some dye batches. Interpretation of the results may not, however, be as straightforward as was once hoped.

➤ Obtaining and keeping reliable reagents

1. Do not use dye samples labeled Alcian Blue 5G or 7G. Only use Alcian Blue 8G samples that dissolve in water to at least 5%. Use Alcian Blue 8GX samples where available.

2. Use the salty solutions immediately following preparation. Do not use samples that precipitate from fresh, 1% pH 5.7 acetate buffered aqueous solutions containing 2 M magnesium chloride.

Individual staining procedures

3. If you have persistent trouble that you attribute to dye impurities, and if no satisfactory dye sample can be found, as a last resort look in Horobin & Goldstein (1972) for analytical and purification suggestions.

▶ Useful routine control procedures

1. Retain a sample of a successful Alcian Blue batch, and use this as a reagent control if doubtful staining occurs.

PROBLEMS AND HOW TO DEAL WITH THEM

▶ Stain or staining solution not as expected

1. If the dye is not readily soluble, or if it rapidly precipitates from the salty solution, check the dye label. Do not use samples labeled Alcian Blue 5G or 7G, as they precipitate easily from salty solutions; and discard unstable dye batches, however they are labeled.

▶ Tissue stains unexpectedly weakly

1. Some dye batches precipitate from high-salt content solutions, especially during the recommended 8-h staining period of this method. So check the dye solution for the presence of precipitate during and after staining, since some batches precipitate completely after half an hour or so.

2. After embedding in water-miscible resins such as glycolmethacrylate, target materials enclosed within the resin section may fail to stain, due to occlusion. Try cutting thinner resin sections, or using paraffin sections.

▶ Unexpected structures stain

1. Strong background staining in low-salt content solutions may reflect too little magnesium chloride. Check for weighing errors due to the deliquescent nature of the salt.

2. Have staining intensities increased in salty dye-baths, when you expected them to decrease? This can certainly

happen, although explanations for the phenomenon vary. Compare staining intensities of differing dye-baths with care. In any event, if intensities rise with salt content, regard any interpretation as suspect.

3. Have staining intensities increased in a low-salt Alcian Blue dye-bath? This may be due to presence of either salt or dextrin impurities. Try another batch of dye or, if all else fails, look in Horobin & Goldstein (1972) for analytical and purification suggestions.

Background reading

For an optimistic account of the critical electrolyte method see the review by its originator (Scott 1973); and for a concise 'consumers' guide' see Scott & Mowry (1970). For more skeptical views see Goldstein & Horobin (1974) and Tas (1977). As an indication of the variety of ways in which impurities of Alcian Blue can influence critical electrolyte concentration staining, see Horobin & Goldstein (1972).

3 Alcian Blue–periodic acid–Schiff (PAS) method for acid and neutral mucin

Background information

In this sequence stain, the acid mucins (e.g. anionic glycosaminoglycans) are first colored by Alcian Blue. Subsequent PAS staining results in contrasting coloration of neutral mucins (e.g. glycoproteins).

The Alcian Blue – a large, hydrophilic cationic dye – is applied from an acid solution, and at a low ionic strength. The dye's large conjugated system results in a high degree of dye aggregation in solution. (*Note*: In this entry, 'Alcian Blue' stands for any of the variant dyes (i.e. Alcian Blue 5G, 7G or 8G), since all are suitable for the present procedure.) Binding of Alcian Blue by anionic glycosaminoglycans is largely due to the van der Waals attractions between Alcian Blue and the tissue components.

Selectivity for tissue anions is due to the cationic charge on the dye. Selectivity for mucins is rate controlled, since the mucin stains more rapidly than nuclear DNA, and very much more rapidly than ribosomal RNA.

The PAS procedure, and its staining mechanism, is described in Entry 38, p. 154.

See Plate 1.

Alcian Blue–periodic acid–Schiff (PAS) method for acid and neutral mucin

Common variants

Some workers have used a 'reversed' staining sequence, i.e. PAS–Alcian Blue rather than Alcian Blue–PAS, or consider both sequences equally effective. However, the reversed sequence has been shown to give rise to positive staining artifacts.

AVOIDING PROBLEMS

➤ What types of specimen processing are suitable?

The method can be applied to paraffin or cryosections; and, for structures such as cartilage matrix or goblet cell mucin, to tissue embedded in water-miscible resins such as glycolmethacrylate. There appear to be no particular fixative restrictions.

➤ Is this procedure easy to carry out?

This procedure is straightforward in practical use.

➤ Obtaining and keeping reliable reagents

1. Reject Alcian Blue samples that are not easily soluble, or that precipitate rapidly.

2. If you have persistent problems that may be due to Alcian Blue impurities, and if no satisfactory dye sample can be found, as a last resort look for analytical and purification suggestions (e.g. Horobin & Goldstein 1972).

3. For comments on obtaining and retaining effective Schiff reagent, see Entry 38, p. 156.

➤ Useful routine control procedures

1. Retain a sample of a successful Alcian Blue batch, and use this as a reagent control if doubtful staining occurs.

2. For comments on controls for use with the PAS segment, see Entry 38, p. 156.

PROBLEMS AND HOW TO DEAL WITH THEM

Note: Only problems peculiar to the Alcian Blue–PAS sequence stain are discussed here. For advice on routine problems arising with the PAS stage of this method, see Entry 38, p. 154.

➤ Stain or staining solution not as expected

1. If Alcian Blue is not readily soluble, or if it rapidly precipitates from solution, discard dye batch.

➤ Tissue stains unexpectedly weakly

1. If, in paraffin sections, structures expected to be alcianophilic do not stain, try extending the hydration step during the de-waxing process, as some alcianophilic structures hydrate rather slowly.

2. After embedding in water-miscible resins such as glycolmethacrylate, alcianophilic target materials enclosed within the resin section may fail to stain due to occlusion (see Gerrits et al 1990). Try cutting thinner resin sections, or using paraffin sections.

➤ Unexpected structures stain

1. High Alcian Blue background staining may be due to presence of either salt or dextrin impurities in the dye. Try another batch of dye.

2. Routinely nonalcianophilic basophilic structures, such as cell nuclei, sometimes stain blue. The causes of this include the following:

    (a) Overlengthy staining, check the Alcian Blue staining time.

    (b) Pretreatment with reagents that increase staining rate, e.g. enzyme extractions, or blockades using extremes of pH. Check if such were used, and, if so, be sceptical.

3. If structures expected to stain with PAS instead stain with

Alcian Blue, check that the staining sequence used was indeed Alcian Blue–PAS, and not PAS–Alcian Blue, as periodate oxidation can generate alcianophilic materials (Johannes & Klessen 1984).

Background reading

The importance of staining rate, and thus of staining time and of various pretreatments, for the selectivity of the low-salt, acidic Alcian Blue method for acid mucins, was demonstrated by Goldstein & Horobin (1974) and Tas (1977).

# Aldehyde Fuchsin for elastic fibers and pancreatic β cells

Background information

Satisfactory Aldehyde Fuchsin can only be prepared from pararosanilin, or from Basic Fuchsin samples rich in that dye. Aldehyde Fuchsin is formed when this dye reacts with acetaldehyde, usually generated from paraldehyde in acidic aqueous ethanol. Purple Schiff bases formed initially are the effective staining compounds. On standing, these transform into various bluish *N*-ethylated basic dyes, plus greenish basic dyes of uncertain structure. A further feature of aging is the continuous precipitation of Aldehyde Fuchsin.

Staining procedures are usually progressive and single-step. Variant methods utilizing a prestaining oxidation step may require poststaining differentiation.

The affinity of Aldehyde Fuchsin for elastic fibers is due to van der Waals attractions between the extended conjugated systems of the Schiff bases, present in Aldehyde Fuchsin, and the hydrophobic protein elastin. It is not clear what underlies the affinity of Aldehyde Fuchsin for pancreatic β-cell granules in unoxidized sections. Staining of oxidized sections is probably due to basic dyeing of sulfonic acids, generated from the sulfur-rich proteins of the secretion granules.

Aldehyde Fuchsin is highly selective, with only β-cell granules, elastin and a few high-affinity basophilic sites (mast cell granules and cartilage matrix) staining. This is due to the salty, acidic ethanolic solution suppressing the binding of Aldehyde Fuchsin to low-affinity basophilic sites such as mucins and nuclei.

See Plate 2.

Common variants

These include: rapidly ripened variants, in which the initial reaction is accelerated by heating or use of high concentrations of reactants, or both; and precipitated Aldehyde Fuchsins, which can be stored indefinitely as dry powders. The staining solutions may be acidified either with hydrochloric or acetic acid. There is some indication that the variants do not all contain the same colored constituents.

AVOIDING PROBLEMS

➤ **What types of specimen processing are suitable?**

There appear to be no fixative limitations. The method can be applied to paraffin and cryosections. However, specimens embedded in hydrophilic resin are unsuitable, as intense background staining of the resin can obscure the specimen.

➤ **Is this procedure easy to carry out?**

The method is straightforward to use with paraffin and cryosections.

➤ **Obtaining and keeping reliable reagents**

1. Use fresh paraldehyde and pararosanilin-rich dye to prepare the stain.

2. Aldehyde Fuchsin working solutions are usually stable for many weeks or even months in the cold, so store in the refrigerator.

3. Occasionally, a batch will precipitate or age rapidly. See below for tips on recognizing such samples.

4. Alternatively, prepare batches of solid Aldehyde Fuchsin, e.g. by the method of Gabe (Kiernan 1990: 129), which are stable in dry form for at least 2 years, and from which working solutions may be prepared in a matter of minutes.

➤ **Useful routine control procedures**

1. Satisfactory Aldehyde Fuchsin batches and procedures should stain pancreatic β cells without prior oxidation, so use such unoxidized sections as positive controls.

PROBLEMS AND HOW TO DEAL WITH THEM

➤ **Stain or staining solution not as expected**

1. If Aldehyde Fuchsin solutions remain red, rather than changing to purple, the paraldehyde may have decomposed. Use a fresh paraldehyde batch or, if this is not available, try doubling the concentration of this reactant.

2. Greenish-blue staining solutions, or the presence of large amounts of purple precipitate when solutions are filtered suggest overaged Aldehyde Fuchsin. Use a fresh batch of stain.

➤ **Tissue stains unexpectedly weakly**

1. Check if Aldehyde Fuchsin has either failed to form, or has overripened. For suggestions on how to make these judgments, see above.

2. Failure of staining of unoxidized sections with a freshly prepared solution of Aldehyde Fuchsin occurs if the stain was prepared from a Basic Fuchsin low in pararosanilin. Use another batch of Aldehyde Fuchsin, prepared from the appropriate dye.

➤ **Unexpected structures stain**

1. If staining of basophilic sites such as mucous goblet cells and nuclei occurs, there may be insufficient electrolyte

present. Check the stain preparation procedure, or try adding extra acid to the stain.

2. Background staining tends to be raised after fixation in dichromate containing agents, perhaps due to oxidation of protein sulfur yielding basophilic groups. Try to avoid using such fixatives.

3. Intense background staining can occur when tissues are embedded in resins such as the glycolmethacrylates (Horobin et al 1991). Due to the slightly lipophilic nature of these resins, this may be inescapable, but try differentiating in acid alcohol.

Background reading

The importance of pararosanilin in preparing effective Aldehyde Fuchsin has been demonstrated by Mowry et al (1980). The chemistry of Aldehyde Fuchsin has been discussed by Proctor & Horobin (1983), and the basis of its selectivity by Horobin (1988: 90). A recent general summary of these topics has been made by Kiernan (1990: 128).

5 Alizarin Red for calcium

Background information

Alizarin Red S is a small, hydrophilic acid dye with indicator properties, one acid–base endpoint being around pH 5. The dye forms coordination complexes with various metal ions. This phenomenon is generally considered to underlie staining of calcium deposits, although it has been suggested that such staining involves the formation of insoluble calcium salts.

One factor influencing sensitivity of staining is pH. Dye–calcium reactivity increases as staining solutions become more alkaline, perhaps because both free calcium ions and ionized phenolic groups are required for complex formation. In any event, the dye–calcium product is solubilized below pH 4. Sensitivity also depends on reaction time, as the dye–calcium complex is formed relatively slowly.

Selectivity is influenced by the same two factors. Use of higher pH solutions inhibits acid dyeing of tissue proteins by Alizarin Red. Diffusion of the reaction product can occur, as it is very slightly soluble under staining conditions and does not have high substantivity for the tissue. Consequently, long staining times lead to poor localization. The resulting conflict between optimum conditions for sensitivity and optimum conditions for localization makes compromise on staining times necessary.

Common variants

Dye concentrations, the pH of staining solutions, staining times, composition of poststaining rinses, and dehydration agents and times all vary between the various recommended methods.

AVOIDING PROBLEMS

▶ **What types of specimen processing are suitable?**

This method is routinely carried out on neutral buffered formalin fixed paraffin or frozen sections. Alcoholic fixatives have been recommended for maximum sensitivity. Acidic fixatives and pretreatments must be avoided. Since the dye ions of Alizarin Red are small and hydrophilic, there should be no serious problems in staining specimens embedded in hydrophilic resins such as glycolmethacrylate.

▶ **Is this procedure easy to carry out?**

This stain is straightforward with paraffin sections, albeit with the sensitivity/selectivity conflict noted above. Consequently, optimum staining times must be determined for individual specimens when demonstrating low calcium concentrations. Often this calls for staining with microscopic control.

▶ **Obtaining and keeping reliable reagents**

1. Avoid impure dyes; see below for tips on recognizing such batches.

2. Weakly acidic Alizarin Red S solutions may often be re-used over a period of several weeks, but avoid contamination by alcohol.

▶ **Useful routine control procedures**

1. Carry out the staining method on a decalcified serial section, e.g. stain after extraction with 1% aqueous HCl for

20 min. Any staining seen after this treatment is unlikely to be due to calcium.

PROBLEMS AND HOW TO DEAL WITH THEM

➤ Stain or staining solution not as expected

1. Yellowish neutral aqueous dye solutions suggest the presence of impurities, which would give unwanted background staining. Use a different, and less yellow, dye batch.

➤ Tissue stains unexpectedly weakly

1. Much tissue calcium is easily lost into aqueous media, including fixative solutions. Try reducing exposure to aqueous fixatives, or use alcoholic fixatives, e.g. Carnoy's fluid; or use cryosections floated directly onto the staining solution.

2. Conversely, some calcium is too tightly bound in the tissue to permit staining. Consider using staining variants with higher pH solutions (see Kashiwa & House 1964, Puchtler et al 1969).

3. Staining intensity is markedly time dependent, so try extending the staining time.

4. The Alizarin Red–calcium reaction product is unstable or soluble below about pH 4. So check the pH of the staining solution and, if low, adjust appropriately.

5. The Alizarin Red–calcium product may be extracted from the stained specimen:

   (a) into poststaining aqueous washes, especially if acidic, so keep acid washes short, and do not leave stained sections standing in (usually slightly acidic) distilled water;

   (b) into alcoholic dehydrating solvents, so keep dehydration times short, or use acetone instead of alcohol.

➤ Unexpected structures stain

1. Background staining can arise due to calcium ions deriving from fixative, so check that the fixative composition is free of calcium.

2. Background coloration, especially after staining for longer times or at lower pH, can also be due to acid dyeing of tissue proteins. Try shortening staining times, check the pH of the staining solution and adjust upwards if necessary, or increase poststaining differentiation/washing times.

3. Diffuse staining of calcium deposits results from diffusion of the dye–calcium product during longer staining times used to detect low calcium concentrations. If this is suspected, try shorter staining times.

4. Is there poor calcium–tissue contrast after treatment with a nuclear counterstain? Toluidine Blue can bind to the Alizarin Red–calcium product, so try another basic dye, such as Methylene Blue.

➤ Staining is of an unexpected color

1. Is background staining yellow? This can result from dye impurities, especially if a low pH method is being used. Try using a higher pH staining variant, and/or a purer batch of dye.

Background reading

For a discussion of the possible role of precipitation, rather than chelation, as a binding mechanism, see Puchtler et al (1969). Factors influencing sensitivity of calcium staining are discussed by Kashiwa & House (1964). Issues underlying the troubleshooting of Alizarin Red methods are considered in papers by Kashiwa & Park (1967), Magee-Russell (1958) and Puchtler et al (1969). The size and hydrophilicity criteria underlying successful staining of hydrophilic resins such as glycolmethacrylate, have been discussed (Gerrits et al 1990, Horobin et al 1991).

6 Adenosine triphosphatase (ATPase) demonstration using calcium–cobalt for fiber typing

Background information

These procedures require adenosine triphosphate (ATP) as the substrate, plus a variety of organic and inorganic salts for buffering and ion capture.

This metal salt precipitation method is based on the selective enzymic hydrolysis of ATP by ATPase, and the subsequent trapping of the inorganic phosphate released by precipitation with calcium ions. This precipitate is converted, by treatment with a cobalt salt, into cobalt phosphate. The cobalt ions are then visualized by treatment with ammonium sulfide, giving rise to a final colored reaction product of cobalt sulfide. The method is made selective for different skeletal muscle fiber types by pretreating and incubating at a variety of pH values.

See Plate 3.

Common variants

The final cobalt sulfide reaction product is an ionic crystal of low solubility in aqueous or organic media. Hence variants are available for mounting in diverse media.

AVOIDING PROBLEMS

➤ **What types of specimen processing are suitable?**

These methods require cryosections.

ATPase demonstration using calcium–cobalt for fiber typing

➤ **Is this procedure easy to carry out?**

This method can be capricious, it is important to check the buffer solutions for precipitate.

➤ **Obtaining and keeping reliable reagents**

1. Some commercial samples of ATP contain significant amounts of adenosine diphosphate (ADP) and inorganic phosphate. Discard such materials.

2. The rate of decomposition of ATP is several percent per month at room temperature, so store ATP samples under refrigeration.

3. The ammonium sulfide working solution must be fresh and not exhibit a deep yellow color.

➤ **Useful routine control procedures**

1. When other phosphatases are present and active at the pH of incubation, ATPase may be selectively inactivated by *p*-chloromercuribenzoate (2.5 mM).

2. Alternatively, since ATPase exhibits relatively high substrate selectivity, incubate in glycerophosphate instead of ATP.

PROBLEMS AND HOW TO DEAL WITH THEM

➤ **Tissue stains unexpectedly weakly**

1. ATPase is substantially inactivated by formaldehyde. So, if formalin fixation was used, try using cold fixation, or use fresh cryosections.

2. Since ADP acts as a competative inhibitor of myosin ATPase, and since commercial samples of ATP may contain significant amounts of ADP, especially after storage, check that your ATP is freshly purchased and prepared.

3. The precipitate of the phosphate intermediate reaction product can dissolve in water, so ensure that postincubation washing is carried out in solutions containing calci-

um ions. Indeed, if necessary, treat the section in 1% aqueous calcium chloride for 5 min prior to incubation in substrate.

➤ Unexpected structures stain

1. Background staining can arise from a failure to remove unprecipitated cobalt ions from the section. So make sure that you wash well following incubation in the cobalt salt.

2. In particular, be suspicious of staining of hyaline granules, hemosiderin, melanin or indeed calcium phosphate, since these structures have a particular affinity for cobalt ions.

Background reading

Some account of the relevant biochemistry, suitable for an understanding of the histochemical method, is provided by Chayen & Bitensky (1991). The application and misapplication of the histochemical method, to paraphrase Firth, has been well reviewed by Brooke & Kaiser (1974), Tunnell & Hart (1977) and Dubowitz (1985).

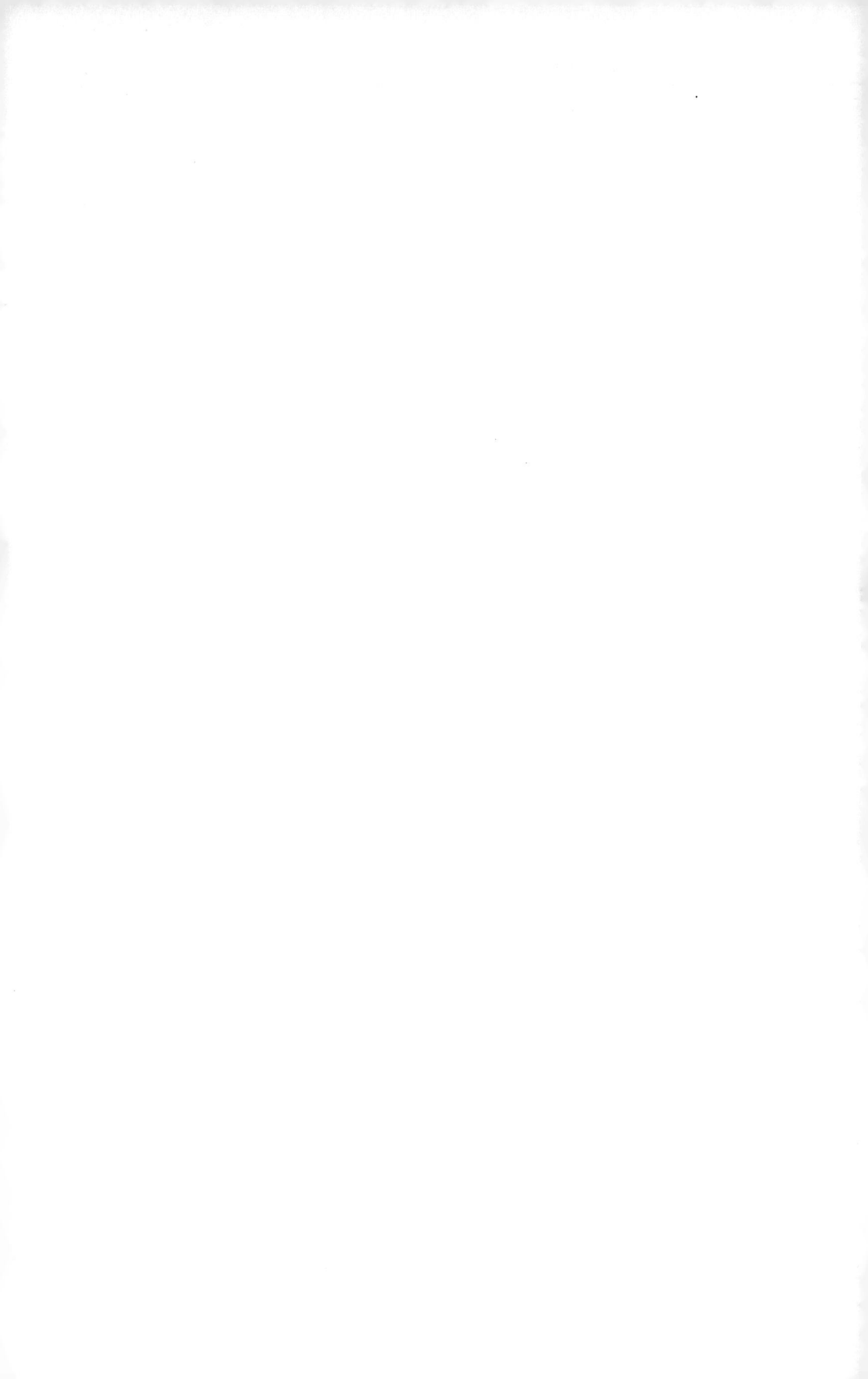

7 Azodye methods for acid phosphatase

Background information

These methods require two reagents: a synthetic organic phosphate substrate, and a diazonium salt visualizing agent. Routinely the substrate is either α-naphthyl phosphate, AS-BI naphthyl phosphate, or a reagent related to the latter. The latter two substrates have larger conjugated systems and are commonly more hydrophobic than the α-naphthol. Routine diazonium salts are Fast Garnet GBC or Hexazotized Pararosanilin, the latter having a relatively large conjugated system.

The azodye procedures demonstrate acid phosphatases selectively by incubating the specimen in substrate at low pH, other phosphatases then being inactive. The enzymically generated, colorless, arylhydroxy reaction product formed as a result of this is visualized by conversion into an insoluble azodye, by reaction with the diazonium salt. Precise tissue or cellular localization of stain, and resistance to extraction into solvents and mountants, is favored by use of reagents with larger conjugated systems (i.e. the AS naphthyl phosphates and Hexazotized Pararosanilin), since this enhances product–tissue protein binding. Precipitation of products is also aided by their being hydrophobic, although this can lead to lipid staining.

See Plate 4.

Common variants

A wide variety of substrates and diazonium salts have been used, providing final stains of a variety of colors. The most common choices of α-naphthyl versus AS naphthyl phosphates, and of Fast Garnet versus Hexazotized Pararosanilin diazonium salts both largely amount to cheapness, purity and simplicity versus technical superiority.

Aqueous mountants are needed for dyes deriving from α-naphthyl phosphate and Fast Garnet; but use of AS naphthyl phosphates plus Hexazotized Pararosanilin permits the use of resin mountants, with resulting benefits in image quality.

Variant methods involve the substrate and visualizing agent being applied sequentially (postcoupling) or being present in one solution (simultaneous coupling). The latter is a much simpler method, but is more susceptible to diazonium salt inhibition of the enzyme, and to conflict between pH requirements of the enzyme and of the coupling reaction.

AVOIDING PROBLEMS

➤ What types of specimen processing are suitable?

Although unfixed cryosections have been used, fixation in a variety of media is routine, enhancing the final specimen morphology. The procedure can be carried out on cryosections, and on specimens embedded in glycolmethacrylate resin, but not on paraffin sections.

➤ Is this procedure easy to carry out?

Except for Hexazotized Pararosanilin, which needs to be prepared freshly, all the routine reagents are simple to obtain and use. In resin it may be necessary to extend staining times.

➤ Obtaining and keeping reliable reagents

1. The α-naphthyl phosphate is often purer, as well as cheaper, than the AS naphthyl phosphates.

Individual staining procedures

2. Commercial batches of diazonium ('fast') salts contain stabilizer, and can be stored long-term in the refrigerator. However, prepare solutions of Hexazotized Pararosanilin freshly for each investigation. In addition, ensure that sodium nitrite solutions used for diazotization are freshly prepared from recently opened containers.

▶ **Useful routine control procedures**

1. Staining should be totally prevented by enzyme inactivation (heat in boiling water for 10 min), or by omitting the substrate from the incubation solution.

2. Staining can be inhibited by addition of sodium fluoride (1–10 mM), copper ions (0.2 mM copper sulphate) or sodium tartrate (10 mM). (*Note*: (a) The use of fluoride for this purpose has been criticized (Chayen & Bitensky, 1991: 91), and (b) such inhibition is organ-dependent.)

PROBLEMS AND HOW TO DEAL WITH THEM

▶ **Stain or staining solution not as expected**

1. When preparing the Hexazotized Pararosanilin the solution should go yellow soon after adding the sodium nitrite. If instead it goes brown or (at any subsequent point in the procedure) red, then try another batch of pararosanilin, or a new jar of sodium nitrite.

▶ **Tissue stains unexpectedly weakly**

1. Overfixation, or use of strongly denaturing agents such as glutaraldehyde, can inhibit acid phosphatase. Try shortening the fixation time, or changing the agent.

2. Diazonium salts can inactivate enzymes, so if you suspect this use Hexazotized Pararosanilin, which is considered to be less inhibitory.

3. The stabilizers present in certain batches of fast salts are also enzyme inhibitory. So try another batch of fast salt,

from a different source, preferably one stated to be stabilized by a different counter ion.

4. Some azodye final reaction products can be extracted into organic solvents or mountants. Try using Hexazotized Pararosanilin as visualizing agent. If you already are using this diazonium salt, ensure that the passage through the graded alcohols to xylene is rapid, and avoid contamination of alcohols by xylene, to minimize dye loss.

➤ Unexpected structures stain

1. If the observed staining is general, whilst well-localized (e.g. punctate) staining was expected, check if Hexazotized Pararosanilin was used as visualizing agent. If not, try this diazonium salt. If you are already using it, try increasing the concentration of salt, but in this case beware enzyme inhibition.

2. Generalized background staining can also arise if incubated sections are washed and stored in water, due to enzymically catalyzed reaction of residual substrate and coupler. Try using more rapid mounting, or alternatively wash in ethanol following incubation to inhibit the enzyme.

3. Staining of lipids or lipid-rich materials can occur when hydrophobic naphthols are used. In such circumstances, try using a more hydrophilic naphthol, or alternatively extract the section with a lipid solvent (e.g. hot chloroform–methanol) prior to staining. Since this staining is nonenzymic, it will also be detected by routine control procedure 1 (see above).

4. Sulphated glycosaminoglycans (e.g. those in mucus goblet cells) may give false-positive staining due to binding of diazonium salts. This is nonenzymic, and so will be detected by routine control procedure 1 (see above).

➤ Staining is of an unexpected color

1. Diazonium salts can react with tissue proteins. Thus,

with Hexazotized Pararosanilin yellow background staining can arise, especially if high pH values or high salt concentrations are used. Try reducing either or both.

Background reading

Some account of the biochemistry, appropriate for understanding the histochemical method, is given by Chayen & Bitensky (1991). More details, including the application of the method, may be found in the books by Bach & Baker (1991), Filipe & Lake (1990) and Pearse & Stoward (1991).

8 Azodye methods for alkaline phosphatase: simultaneous coupling

Background information

These methods involve a synthetic organic phosphate substrate, plus a diazonium salt as a visualizing agent. Typically, the substrate is either α-naphthyl phosphate or AS-BI naphthyl phosphate, or a reagent related to the latter. The latter two substrates have relatively large conjugated systems and are commonly more hydrophobic. Routinely used diazonium salts include Fast Blue RR or Fast Red TR.

Simultaneous coupling azodye procedures demonstrate alkaline phosphatases selectively by incubating the specimen in substrate under alkaline conditions, where other phosphatases are minimally active. The enzymically generated colorless arylhydroxy reaction product is visualized by converting it to an insoluble azodye, using the diazonium salt. Precise tissue and cellular localization of stain, and resistance to extraction into solvents and mountants, is favored by use of AS naphthyl phosphates, the larger conjugated systems of which enhance product–tissue protein binding. Precipitation of products is also aided by their being hydrophobic, although this can lead to lipid staining.

Common variants

Several substrates and diazonium salts have been recommended, so a variety of final colors is available. The choice between α-naphthyl and AS naphthyl phosphates amounts to cheapness and purity versus superior localization.

AVOIDING PROBLEMS

➤ What types of specimen processing are suitable?

Although unfixed cryosections have been recommended, fixation in formalin and other media prior to cryotomy is commonplace. Moreover, alkaline phosphatase activity in some sites survives even paraffin embedding. Specimens embedded in glycolmethacrylate resin give strong staining plus exceptionally well-localized demonstrations of alkaline phosphatases.

➤ Is this procedure easy to carry out?

The alkaline phosphatases are robust to fixation. All the reagents are easy to obtain and simple to use, although the diazonium salts are unstable once in solution. The AS naphthyl phosphates are rather hydrophobic, and require bringing into solution using an organic solvent before mixing with aqueous buffer. When using resin sections, extended staining times are not required.

➤ Obtaining and keeping reliable reagents

1. The α-naphthyl phosphate is often purer, as well as cheaper, than the AS naphthyl compounds.

2. Commercial diazonium (i.e. 'fast') salts contain stabilizer, and can be stored long-term in the refrigerator. However, prepare the solutions freshly for each stain, since once dissolved the salts quickly deteriorate.

➤ Useful routine control procedures

1. Staining should be totally prevented by enzyme inactivation (heat in boiling water for 10 min), or by omitting the substrate from the incubation solution.

2. A useful inhibitor of alkaline phosphatase activity at

most sites is levamisole (0.1–0.5 mM). To inhibit the intestinal and placental enzyme, L-phenylalanine has often been used.

PROBLEMS AND HOW TO DEAL WITH THEM

> ► **Tissue stains unexpectedly weakly**

1. Some diazonium salts, including Fast Blue RR, are unstable in solution. Make sure the fast salt is dissolved immediately prior to incubating the slide.

2. Penetration of reagents into the specimens can be a rate-controlling step. If unfixed sections were used, try brief fixation, as this can permeabilize the specimen. If an AS naphthyl phosphate was used, try α-naphthyl phosphate, as this is smaller and thus faster diffusing.

3. Azodye final reaction products may be extracted into organic solvents or mountants. Check that the mountant used was aqueous.

> ► **Unexpected structures stain**

1. Staining of lipids or lipid-rich materials can occur when hydrophobic naphthols are used. In such circumstances, try using a more hydrophilic naphthol; alternatively, extract the section with a lipid solvent (e.g. hot chloroform-methanol) prior to staining. Since this artifactual staining is nonenzymic, it will also be detected by routine control procedure 1 (see above).

2. Sulfated glycosaminoglycans (e.g. those in mucus goblet cells) may give false-positive staining due to binding of diazonium salts. This is nonenzymic, and so will be detected by routine control procedure 1 (see above).

> ► **Staining is of an unexpected color**

1. A generalized background staining of a different color to that expected, and perhaps seen, at enzymic sites can

arise from reaction of the diazonium salt with tissue proteins. Ignore such background staining.

Background reading

The biochemical significance of histochemically demonstrable alkaline phosphatase was once disputed. This is no longer so, and for a general review of the biochemistry of the alkaline phosphatases (EC 3.1.3.1) see Butterworth (1983). A critical account of the histochemical methodology has been given by Chayen & Bitensky (1991).

Best's Carmine for glycogen

Background information

The active colorant is carminic acid, a component of the Carmine, which is the usual material used to prepare stock solutions. Carminic acid is a small, hydrophilic anionic dye that readily forms cationic coordination complexes with metal ions such as iron and aluminum.

The working solution of the Best's Carmine stain contains ammonia, potassium carbonate and chloride, and methanol, in addition to the dye. Alkali, electrolyte, methanol and dye are all necessary for effective staining (see below).

When applied as a substantially nonaqueous, high-salt concentration working solution, carminic acid binds to polysaccharides by hydrogen bonding. Background acid dyeing is suppressed by the alkaline and salty environment. Use of a nonaqueous poststaining wash is essential, as water is such an effective hydrogen bonding solvent that it rapidly strips the dye from the biopolymer.

Common variants

Several variants may be found in the literature, and these are not always entirely consistent. For example, Mallory recommended filtration of stock solutions, whereas Bensley forbids it. Other variants use alternative dyes (e.g. haematoxylin and Alizarin Red S), permitting colorations other than red. Periodate oxidation prior to dyeing has been suggested, to make the method more precisely comparable to periodic acid–Schiff (PAS) staining.

AVOIDING PROBLEMS

➤ **What types of specimen processing are suitable?**

This method is routinely applied to formalin-fixed paraffin sections. If used with tissues embedded in hydrophilic resin media such as glycolmethacrylates, section swelling proves a technical difficulty.

➤ **Is this procedure easy to carry out?**

Even with paraffin sections the method is complicated, although it does not involve any technically ambiguous steps.

➤ **Obtaining and keeping reliable reagents**

1. Most commercial dye samples contain sufficient colored material for this method to be carried out successfully, so if one sample proves poor, purchase another. If this strategy fails, and you wish to check dye content, assay using a simple method described by Marshall & Horobin (1974a).

2. Store the stock solution in a dark container in the refrigerator, when it should be reasonably stable for several months.

3. The working solution can be stable for about a week, but it is better to prepare it immediately before use.

➤ **Useful routine control procedures**

1. Stain a section after prior extraction with amylase, after which no glycogen should be present, and so no staining occur.

PROBLEMS AND HOW TO DEAL WITH THEM

➤ Stain or staining solution not as expected

1. Has dye precipitated from the working solution? This can occur if the ammonia evaporates, so keep the working solution in a closed container and filter immediately before use.

2. Does dye precipitate onto the section during the staining process? If so, stain in a closed container, and after staining do not let the sections dry, but wash immediately with alcohol or differentiator.

➤ Tissue stains unexpectedly weakly

1. Glycogen, being a water-soluble polysaccharide, can be extracted from the specimen into aqueous fixatives. Try fixing specimens in picric–formaldehyde (Chayen & Bitensky 1991: 102) or alcoholic media.

2. The stock solution deteriorates with age, so check the age of the stock solution and, if elderly, try lengthening the time of staining.

3. Dye may have been lost by precipitation prior to staining. Keep the dye in a closed container and check working solution for precipitate.

4. Loss of methanol by evaporation reduces staining intensity. Make sure the working solution is freshly prepared, and is stored and used in a closed container.

5. Sections inadvertently washed in water following staining, rather than in differentiator or alcohol, de-stain extremely rapidly, so check the nature of the washing solution used.

➤ Unexpected structures stain

1. In the absence of a nuclear counterstain, cell nuclei are often stained. This is probably due to a contaminating cationic iron–carminic acid coordination complex, so ignore this artifact.

Background reading

An account of the underlying physicochemical basis of this stain is available (Horobin & Murgatroyd 1971).

10 Chloroacetate esterase for mast and myeloid cells

Background information

These methods require two key reagents: a synthetic organic phosphate and a diazonium salt visualizing agent. Routinely, the substrate is naphthol AS D chloroacetate, which has a relatively large conjugated system and is somewhat hydrophobic. Routine diazonium salts are Fast Blue RR or Hexazotized Pararosanilin, the latter having a relatively large conjugated system.

The procedure demonstrates the chymotrypsin-like proteases present in mast cells and the more differentiated myeloid cell lines. The selectivity depends on the relatively rapid hydrolysis of the naphthylchloroacetate ester by these enzymes. Visualization of the colorless, arylhydroxy hydrolysis product is achieved by its conversion into an insoluble azodye, using a diazonium salt.

Precise cellular localization of stain, and resistance to extraction into solvents and mountants, is favored by use of reagents with larger conjugated systems (i.e. the AS naphthol and Hexazotized Pararosanilin), as this enhances product–tissue protein binding. Precipitation of the intermediate reaction product is also aided by its being hydrophobic.

See Plate 5.

Common variants

Diazonium salt visualizing agents may be a stabilized fast salt, routinely Fast Blue RR, or freshly prepared Hexazotized Pararosanilin. When the latter is used sections can be mounted in resin, otherwise an aqueous mountant is required.

AVOIDING PROBLEMS

➤ **What types of specimen processing are suitable?**

Frozen sections or formalin-fixed paraffin sections can be used. The method is also applied to blood smears, fixed in formaldehyde vapor.

➤ **Is this procedure easy to carry out?**

The enzyme concerned is robust, and hence fixed or unfixed material, or even paraffin processed specimens, can be used. If the latter are used, long incubation times are required. Preparation of the working solution of Fast Blue RR is simple, but this visualizing agent necessitates using an aqueous mountant. Preparation of Hexazotized Pararosanilin is more troublesome, but permits mounting in superior, resin systems. The substrate, chloroacetate derivative of naphthol AS D, is rather hydrophobic and requires initial solubilization in an organic solvent such as acetone or dimethylformamide. Be prepared for the color of the incubating solution to be whitish pink before filtration.

➤ **Useful routine control procedures**

1. Staining should be totally prevented by enzyme inactivation (heat in boiling water for 10 min) or by omitting the substrate from the incubation solution.

2. This esterase, especially in myeloid cells, is inhibited by phytostigmine (1 mM), taurocholate (10 mM) and diisopropyl fluorophosphate (10 mM).

PROBLEMS AND HOW TO DEAL WITH THEM

▶ Obtaining and keeping reliable reagents

Commercial diazonium (i.e. 'fast') salts contain stabilizer, and can be stored long-term in the refrigerator. However, prepare the solutions freshly for each stain, since once dissolved the salts quickly deteriorate.

▶ Tissue stains unexpectedly weakly

1. With bony specimens needing decalcification, use a short decalcification in EDTA. Use of acidic decalcification schedules can weaken the staining reaction.

2. The diazonium salt Fast Blue RR is unstable in solution. Make sure that this fast salt is dissolved immediately prior to incubating the slide.

3. If you are using paraffin sections, try extending the staining time. Paraffin sections usually require staining times considerably longer than for cryosections.

4. If you are looking for myeloid cells, try extending the staining time. Myeloid cells may require staining times considerably longer than do mast cells.

5. If you are looking at myeloid cells, note that, whilst in general the more mature the myeloid cells the weaker the reaction, myeloblasts may be nonstaining.

▶ Unexpected structures stain

1. If there are deposits of stain on the background tissue, check that the pH of the incubation solution has not risen.

2. Staining of lipids or lipid-rich materials can occur when hydrophobic naphthols are used. In such circumstances, try using a more hydrophilic naphthol; alternatively, extract the section with a lipid solvent (e.g. hot chloroform–methanol) prior to staining. Since this type of staining is nonenzymic, it will also be detected by routine control procedure 1 (see above).

3. Sulphated glycosaminoglycans (e.g. those in mucus goblet cells) may give false-positive staining due to binding of diazonium salts. This is nonenzymic, and so will be detected by routine control procedure 1 (see above).

➤ Staining is of an unexpected color

1. A generalized background staining of a different color to that expected, and perhaps seen, at enzymic sites can arise from reaction of the diazonium salt with tissue proteins. Ignore such background staining.

➤ Nature of staining is unusual

1. When staining blood smears, if coloration is diffuse (i.e. staining localization is poor) check that the specimen was fixed in formaldehyde vapor, not wet fixed in methanol.

Background reading

A good account of the histochemical implications of the rather complex biochemistry of esterases is provided by Chayen & Bitensky (1991). For its uses in pathology, see Bancroft & Stevens (1996).

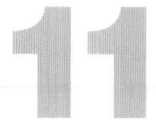

11 Congo Red for amyloid (Highman's method) and related methods

Background information

Congo Red is an anionic bis azodye, with a large conjugated system.

The key staining step in Highman's procedure applies Congo Red from an aqueous alcoholic solution, removing nonspecific background by subsequent differentiation with aqueous alcoholic alkali. Variant methods use a salty, alkaline alcoholic dye solution, pretreat with salty, alkaline alcohol, or differentiate, or merely 'rinse', in aqueous alcohol. Nuclei are counterstained with an aluminium haematoxylin, either before or after the Congo Red step, depending on the variant adopted.

The dye binding to amyloid depends on the use of a dye possessing a large conjugated system, and hence able to attach noncoulombically by means of van der Waals forces. The method's selectivity derives from the dye being anionic, whilst the dye-bath (and/or the prestaining wash, and the poststaining differentiator) are of high pH. This combination inhibits or reverses acid dyeing of most proteins by the Congo Red, as most proteins are themselves anionic under the alkaline conditions used. The overall result is that most proteins fail to stain, amyloid being an exception.

Staining of amyloid by Congo Red has another unusual feature: the bound dye exhibits birefringence when viewed in polarized light.

See Plate 6.

Common variants

There are a number of variations of the Highmans's method, as indicated above. Essentially these constitute trade-offs between minimizing the number of solutions used and the number of components in these solutions, versus avoiding the need for a differentiation step. Other dyes of similar properties (e.g. Sirius Red) have been used instead of Congo Red.

AVOIDING PROBLEMS

➤ **What types of specimen processing are suitable?**

Any type of fixative or section can be used.

➤ **Is this procedure easy to carry out?**

The differentiation step, especially in Highman's procedure, can be tricky for inexperienced workers.

➤ **Obtaining and keeping reliable reagents**

1. Commercial batches of Congo Red seem fairly consistent but not pure, as a yellow monoazo dye is sometimes present as an impurity. No problems relating to impure dye have been reported.

2. Stock dye solution is stable for several weeks.

3. Solutions of Congo Red are not stable in the presence of salt and alkali, so prepare such working solutions freshly.

➤ **Useful routine control procedures**

1. Stain a slide known to contain amyloid as a positive control, along with the unknown.

PROBLEMS AND HOW TO DEAL WITH THEM

➤ **Tissue stains unexpectedly weakly**

1. Weakly stained deposits of amyloid can lose all their Congo Red by overdifferentiation following staining. (*Note*: Describing treatment with solvent as a 'rinse' does not mean that dye will not be lost. If in doubt, underdifferentiate and distinguish nonspecific background by its lack of birefringence in polarized light.)

2. The green birefringence seen in polarized light may not be apparent in thin sections. If birefringence is absent in thin sections, check out a 6 μm section.

➤ **Unexpected structures stain**

1. As well as amyloid, Highman's and related methods will give red or pink staining of the corpora amylacea of brain and prostate, elastic fibers, eosinophil granules, keratin, and even of cellulose (which may be present in animal tissue as a contaminant) and, after some fixatives, of collagen.

2. Indeed, even the birefringence seen when viewing with polarized light has been seen in cellulose, young Haversion bone and, after fixation in alcohol, Bouin's or Carnoy's solution, in connective tissue fibers.

3. When there is generalized pink background staining, either ignore it or check its significance by viewing in polarized light, or lengthen the poststaining rinse or differentiation.

➤ **Staining is of an unexpected color**

1. Generalized yellow background staining can arise from the presence of dye impurity. Ignore this staining.

Background reading

A short account of the basis of amyloid staining by Congo

Red has been given by Kiernan (1990: 180). The nature of the staining by dyes possessing large conjugated systems under high pH, high-salt concentration conditions has been discussed by Horobin & Bennion (1973) and Bennion & Horobin (1974).

Individual staining procedures

12 Cresyl Fast Violet for nucleic acids in nervous tissue

Background information

Cresyl Fast Violet is a weakly lipophilic cationic dye, with a conjugated system of moderate size. A related but more hydrophilic dye, Cresyl Violet, is often substituted in this procedure. Indeed, some commercial samples labeled Cresyl Fast Violet have been found to be Cresyl Violet.

The staining procedure involves the basic dyeing of the nucleic acid polyanions present in nuclei, nucleoli and Nissl substance of neurons, neuroglia and endothelial cells. Selectivity of staining is due to the dye being cationic. Dye binding is aided by van der Waals attractions; as shown by the resistance of Cresyl Fast Violet (and indeed Cresyl Violet) to extraction into ethanolic dehydrating fluids. Alternative Nissl stains such as Neutral Red and Thionin have smaller conjugated systems, and the consequent lesser van der Waals attractions and looser binding require dehydration in acetone or butanol, not ethanol.

Selective staining is routinely achieved by means of differentiation. This is often necessitated due to the use of thick sections in neuroanatomical investigations. Sometimes acetic acid is added to the working solution, to suppress nuclear staining whilst retaining Nissl staining.

Common variants

This is a classic method with many variants, especially with regard to the time of and solvents used for differentiation. In part this reflects the routine application of this method to thick sections. However, the ambiguity surrounding the chemical identity of the dye involved has doubtless also played a role in multiplying procedures.

AVOIDING PROBLEMS

➤ What types of specimen processing are suitable?

The method is routinely applied to alcohol, Carnoy's solution or neutral formol fixed paraffin sections. Staining may also be carried out on specimens embedded in water-miscible resins, such as the glycolmethacrylates.

➤ Is this procedure easy to carry out?

Staining is straightforward with paraffin sections, but differentiation under microscopic control may not be. Standardization is not always possible, and the procedure can be fiddly. With tissues embedded in hydrophilic resin media such as glycolmethacrylates, high background staining has been reported by some workers; this is not surprising given the lipophilic nature of the dye.

➤ Obtaining and keeping reliable reagents

1. Satisfactory Cresyl Fast Violet samples are available commercially. However, as noted above, errors of dye identity can arise. If all else fails, check dye identities spectroscopically using published spectra (see Lillie 1977, Green 1990).

2. Filter the working solution before use. At least for some variants, the working solution should not be re-used.

PROBLEMS AND HOW TO DEAL WITH THEM

➤ Stain or staining solution not as expected

1. If a new batch of dye proves difficult to dissolve, you may be using real Cresyl Fast Violet for the first time,

whereas in the past you have been supplied with mislabeled Cresyl Violet. Fear not, and continue.

➤ Tissue stains unexpectedly weakly

1. The method involves differentiation, and it is possible to overdifferentiate. This is particularly true when working with thick sections. Depending on the variant used, try shortening exposure to alcohols, or dehydrate in nonethanolic media, or omit use of cajuput oil, and so on.

➤ A 'quantitative' staining artifact

1. Cells in the middle layer of thick sections may fail to stain. However, this will not be obvious if the cells in the outer layers stain well (Cooper et al 1988). So, in quantitative work, compare cell counts after varying staining times, and beware increases in cell numbers with increases in time. If this does occur, try longer staining times, avoid low dye concentrations and, if possible, avoid thick sections.

➤ Unexpected structures stain

1. High background staining can occur, especially with thick sections. Try extending or repeating the differentiation.

2. High background staining can occur with tissues embedded in hydrophilic resin media such as glycolmethacrylates. Try differentiation in ethanolic solutions, but beware excessive loss of stain and wrinkling of the section.

Background reading

For an account of how the chemical structure of this dye has in the past been confused, and the nature of the products supplied commercially erratic, see Green (1990: 235) and Lillie (1977: 412). The hydrophilicity criteria underlying successful staining of hydrophilic resins, such as glycolmethacrylate, has been discussed (Horobin et al 1991).

13 Fast Green for basic proteins

Background information

Fast Green FCF is a hydrophilic, anionic dye of moderate size. Binding of dye to protein is aided by van der Waals attractions due to the stain's extended conjugated system. Selectivity is controlled by the electric charges carried by dye and tissue substrates, as the anionic dye only attaches to cationic substrates. At the alkaline pH of the working solution, only basic (i.e. arginine and lysine-rich) proteins stain, since only these proteins still carry an overall positive charge.

Since selectivity is so strongly dependent on the electric charge of the substrate, presence of high concentrations of tissue polyanions will inhibit staining. Consequently, as the method is most commonly used for staining nuclear histones, a DNA extraction step precedes dyeing.

Common variants

Both hot trichloracetic acid solution and DNase have been recommended to extract the DNA.

AVOIDING PROBLEMS

➤ **What types of specimen processing are suitable?**

For qualitative work the method does not require any particular fixative, although for quantitative work various fixatives have been recommended. The method is routinely applied to paraffin sections, although specimens embedded in hydrophilic resin media such as glycolmethacrylates can also be used.

▶ Is this procedure easy to carry out?

The method is straightforward to use with paraffin sections. When applied to sections of hydrophilic resins such as glycolmethacrylates, high background staining has been found by some workers. This is not surprising, given the moderate size of the dye.

▶ Obtaining and keeping reliable reagents

1. Commercial samples are typically of high and uniform purity, perhaps reflecting the onetime use of Fast Green as a food dye.

▶ Useful control procedures

1. To check the efficacy of the DNA extraction step, replace the extraction by a water control. Staining should now be weaker.

2. To check that stained material is protein, use specimens treated with trypsin prior to staining.

PROBLEMS AND HOW TO DEAL WITH THEM

▶ Tissue stains unexpectedly weakly

1. Weak staining of specimens fixed in acidic media may be due to extraction of protein, try fixing in alcohol or formalin.

2. When the method is used to demonstrate nuclear histones, staining is inhibited by the presence of DNA. Pale staining may indicate ineffective extraction. Check by using control procedure 1 (see above).

▶ Unexpected structures stain

1. Background staining of the resin may occur when the

method is applied to specimens embedded in hydrophilic resin media, such as glycolmethacrylates, which resist aqueous extraction. Try differentiating in ethanolic solutions.

Background reading

A modern account of this method has been given by James & Tas (1984). The size criteria underlying successful staining of hydrophilic resins, such as glycolmethacrylate, has been discussed (Gerrits et al 1990).

Individual staining procedures

14 Feulgen stain for DNA

Background information

Key reagents in the Feulgen nucleal staining procedure are the acid used for hydrolysis, and Schiff reagent. This latter is a solution containing a colorless derivative of Basic Fuchsin, in which a sulfite moiety has been attached to the central carbon atom. Satisfactory Schiff reagent can be prepared from either of the commercially available homologs of Basic Fuchsin, i.e. pararosanilin or New Fuchsin. Other necessary components of Schiff reagent are hydrogen ions and sulfite ions.

Feulgen staining involves initial depurination of DNA by acid hydrolysis, yielding apurinic acid. Rearrangement of the deoxyribose moieties follows, yielding aldehyde groups. On exposure to Schiff reagent, these give rise to colorless reaction products, which are converted to magenta final reaction products by the post-Schiff-reagent washing steps.

Sensitivity and selectivity are dependent on several factors. The acid-labile DNA and derived apurinic acid must be retained in the specimen during specimen preparation, acid hydrolysis and staining. DNA is almost the only biopolymer to yield aldehydes following acid hydrolysis. Endogenous aldehyde groups must be absent or their location known. Schiff reagent must not decompose during staining.

See Plate 7.

Common variants

Variants of the Feulgen procedure, whilst all possessing the characteristics alluded to above, differ as follows. Two major variants involve the nature of the acid and the hydrolysis step: use hot 5 M hydrochloric acid for a few minutes, or cold 1 M hydrochloric acid for a longer period. Optimum hydrolysis times are achieved by balancing achieving complete depurination against losing DNA fragments into the solution. With regard to the composition of the Schiff reagent and the nature of staining process, the source and concentration of sulfite and hydrogen ions may vary; bisulfite or metabisulfite plus a mineral acid are routine. The solutions are always strongly acidic, and contain excess sulfite over that needed to react with the Basic Fuchsin. The molar concentrations of this dye are similar in the different methods. The temperatures and times of treatment with Schiff reagent vary.

With regard to the poststaining treatment, both sulfite solutions and running water have been recommended for washing Schiff-treated specimens. Both have disadvantages in quantitative work (see Demalsy & Callebaut 1967, Chayen & Bitensky 1991: 81).

AVOIDING PROBLEMS

▶ What types of specimen processing are suitable?

The method is routinely applied to formalin-fixed paraffin sections. A variety of nonacidic fixatives may be used, but note that fixation has a marked influence on the optimum period of hydrolysis. The procedure may also be carried out on hydrophilic resin media, such as glycolmethacrylates. In resin formulations that are only weakly cross-linked, acidic reagents can cause significant resin swelling, and loss of sections from slides. Cryosections have also been used, with the addition of colloid-stabilizing agents to the hydrolysis and staining solutions.

➤ Is this procedure easy to carry out?

The Feulgen procedure has no significant difficulties for the benchworker using paraffin sections.

➤ Obtaining and keeping reliable reagents

1. At the time of writing, standardized Schiff reagent is not commercially available. However, since a simple procedure for preparing stable, dry Schiff reagent has been published (Galassi 1993) this situation may improve.

2. In the interim, use only colorless batches of Schiff reagent. See below for tips on the recognition of contamination or decomposition.

3. Store Schiff reagent tightly sealed, in a refrigerator.

➤ Useful control procedures

1. Stain a specimen omitting the acid-hydrolysis step. Endogenous or artifactual aldehydes will be colored purple.

2. Insert an aldehyde blockade after the posthydrolysis wash, and before treatment with Schiff reagent (Bancroft & Stevens 1990: 104). Staining of this control indicates staining due to nonaldehyde materials.

PROBLEMS AND HOW TO DEAL WITH THEM

➤ Stain or staining solution not as expected

1. If the Schiff reagent looks yellow-brown, contamination by acridines may have occurred. Use another batch of reagent, or try decolorizing with activated charcoal as in preparation of the reagent.

2. If the Schiff reagent is pink tinged and smells only weakly of sulfur dioxide (care!), it may be overaged, as Basic Fuchsin is slowly formed on standing. Use fresh Schiff reagent, or reconstitute with bisulfite (see Chung & Chen 1970).

▶ **Tissue stains unexpectedly weakly**

1. DNA may be hydrolyzed, and the fragments lost from the specimen, before the Feulgen procedure is even started.

    (a) Acidic aqueous fixatives can have this effect, so avoid long fixations in such media.

    (b) DNA may also be lost into acidic decalcification media, so decalcify in nonacidic media, e.g. EDTA if you wish to follow this by Feulgen staining.

2. DNA may also be over-hydrolyzed, and the fragments lost, during the acid-hydrolysis step. Try shortening the hydrolysis time, or try using a cold-hydrolysis method.

3. Conversely, under-hydrolysis can also give rise to weak staining.

    (a) A mismatch may occur between the fixative used and the hydrolysis time adopted, so check the literature and adjust the hydrolysis time accordingly.

    (b) Under-hydrolysis can also arise with short, hot-hydrolysis methods, so with such procedures you must ensure that the acid is preheated before commencing the hydrolysis.

4. In microwave-accelerated procedures, it is possible to over-hydrolyze and extract apurinic acids, even during the treatment with Schiff reagent. Try shorter times in the Schiff reagent, or abandon microwaving the Schiff treatment step.

5. If the method is being used quantitatively, note that fading may occur. If possible, measure staining intensity immediately following staining, or at least store stained specimens in the dark.

▶ **Unexpected structures stain**

1. Pink background staining may be due to decomposition of Schiff reagent.

Individual staining procedures

(a) This may be due to aging (see above).

(b) It can also arise by thermal decomposition during microwave-accelerated staining. So if the stain becomes transiently pink during hot staining, reduce time or temperature settings on the oven.

2. Pink background staining also occurs due to artifactual tissue aldehyde groups.

   (a) These can arise because of acrolein or glutaraldehyde fixation. Try another fixative, or treat sections with borohydride prior to oxidation (Bancroft & Stevens 1990: 234).

   (b) Alternatively, the problem may be due to insufficient washing of tissue following formaldehyde fixation. Try extending the wash time.

3. Localized purple or red staining of 'nontarget' structures can take place for various reasons.

   (a) Deposits of carbonates and other salts can decompose Schiff reagent. This phenomenon can be detected by routine control procedure 2 (see above).

   (b) Lipid-rich material can generate plasmals following acid hydrolysis, so becoming Schiff-positive. Try extracting the section with chloroform–methanol prior to oxidation, and see if staining is now negative.

▶ **Staining is of an unexpected color**

1. Yellow-brown staining may be due to contamination of Schiff reagent with acridines (see above).

Background reading

The structure and staining mechanism of Schiff reagent is now clear (Nettleton & Carpenter 1977, Robins et al 1980). A demonstration that satisfactory Schiff reagent can be prepared from pararosanilin or New Fuchsin was made by Teichman et al (1980). For a discussion of the key issue of the relative rates of depurination versus loss of DNA fragments during acid hydrolysis, see Andersson & Kjellstrand (1975).

For a discussion of the difficulties involved in standardizing the Feulgen stain, see Schulte & Wittekind (1989). The size and hydrophilicity criteria underlying successful staining of hydrophilic resins, such as glycolmethacrylate, have been discussed (Gerrits et al 1990, Horobin et al 1991). From a general troubleshooting perspective, a valuable account of the Feulgen stain is that given by Chayen & Bitensky (1991).

Individual staining procedures

15 Fouchet technique for liver bile pigments

Background information

The key reagents are ferric chloride, plus strong trichloracetic acid. These are applied directly to the tissue sections, and then washed out in water.

The ferric chloride, under the strongly acidic conditions of use, serves to oxidize bile pigments, forming green biliverdin and blue cholecyanin in bile pigment deposits of all sizes.

See Plate 8.

Common variants

Counterstaining the Fouchet stained section with Van Gieson solution is often carried out.

AVOIDING PROBLEMS

➤ **What types of specimen processing are suitable?**

This method can be used after any fixative, and with cryosections or paraffin sections. It would not be suitable for tissue embedded in water-miscible glycolmethacrylate sections, due to the strongly acidic nature of the staining solution.

➤ **Is this procedure easy to carry out?**

This is a quick and simple method, although it does use an aggressive reagent.

➤ Obtaining and keeping reliable reagents

1. It is advisable to use analytical grade reagents, and to make up the staining solution freshly for each investigation.

➤ Useful routine control procedures

1. Use sections known to contain bile pigments as positive controls. Stain one by the Fouchet procedure, and another by the Fouchet procedure followed by Van Gieson solution.

PROBLEMS AND HOW TO DEAL WITH THEM

➤ Tissue stains unexpectedly weakly

1. If you are looking for bile in the Aschoff–Rokitansky sinuses or in hemorrhagic or infarcted areas, note that this method may fail to stain. Try using the Gmelin or the Stein techniques in these instances.

Background reading

A widely used version of this procedure is that described by Hall (1960).

Individual staining procedures

16 Gimenez method for *Helicobacter pylori*

Background information

This procedure uses two basic dyes, Basic Fuchsin and Malachite Green. These are both cationic dyes, of much the same size, but Malachite Green is more hydrophobic.

The method involves sequence staining of sections. The primary stain is Basic Fuchsin, applied at room temperature from an aqueous alcoholic solution containing phenol, i.e. Carbol Fuchsin. The counterstain is an aqueous solution of Malachite Green. This is applied briefly, and the section washed and inspected, with this cycle being repeated until the section appears blue/green to the naked eye. The section is then blotted, air dried and mounted in resin.

The initial step involving a very concentrated solution of Basic Fuchsin overstains both microorganisms and tissue background. The second dye then replaces the first, with this occurring slowly in the poorly permeable bacteria.

AVOIDING PROBLEMS

➤ **What types of specimen processing are suitable?**

This procedure is routinely carried out on formalin-fixed paraffin sections.

➤ **Is this procedure easy to carry out?**

This method, applied to paraffin sections, is fiddly to carry out due to the need to remove the primary stain from the tissue background without de-staining the bacteria. For this reason, stain only single sections per slide.

➤ Obtaining and keeping reliable reagents

1. Carbol Fuchsin stock solutions are typically stable for months.

2. However, if any substantial amount of dark-red precipitate forms during storage, prepare or obtain a fresh batch of stain.

➤ Useful routine control procedures

1. Retain a specimen containing *Helicobacter*, and take sections from this through the staining procedure as a positive control.

PROBLEMS AND HOW TO DEAL WITH THEM

➤ Tissue stains unexpectedly weakly

1. If no red-stained bacteria are seen in the positive control, then overstaining with Malachite Green may have occurred. Repeat, reducing the exposure to the counterstain.

2. If sections show little or no counterstaining once mounted, although staining of bacteria with the primary dye has occurred, check that stained sections were blotted dry (not washed) and air dried (not taken through the alcohols). Malachite Green is rather hydrophobic, and very alcohol soluble.

➤ Unexpected structures stain

1. If there are numerous irregular red particles present, check if they are deposited on the surface of the section. If so, these are probably particles of precipitated Basic Fuchsin. Remember to filter the primary stain just before use.

Background reading

The original method was described by Gimenez (1964). For its application to the histological demonstration of *Helicobacter*, see McMullenen et al (1987).

17 Gomori's one-step trichrome

Background information

The acid dyes used in the standard variant of this method are Chromotrope 2R, the red anion of which is fairly small and hydrophilic, and Fast Green FCF, the green anion of which is much larger and rather more hydrophilic. A heteropolyacid, phosphotungstic acid, is also used, the anions of which are large. When a nuclear counterstain is used, this will be an aluminium hematoxylin.

These reagents are applied from a single strongly acidic solution, after the prior staining of cell nuclei with an alum hematoxylin. The mixture of acid dyes then gives a polychrome staining without differentiation: collagen stains blue/green; and muscle and other cytoplasms and erythrocytes stain red. If a prior nuclear staining is applied, these organelles will be gray-blue.

The affinity of the acid dyes may be considered as the binding of these anionic compounds to tissue proteins, enhanced by the plentiful cationic substituents present due to the highly acidic dye-bath. Selectivity appears due to rate control, since staining by the large blue-green dye is restricted to the permeable, and so fast staining, collagen fibers, whereas the other, less permeable, structures stain with the smaller red dye. The role of phosphotungstic acid is unclear in the present system.

See Plate 9.

Common variants

Probably the only common variant is the replacement of Fast Green by Light Green SF. However, the latter dye is more prone to fading.

AVOIDING PROBLEMS

➤ What types of specimen processing are suitable?

It is routinely used on paraffin sections, but can also be applied to cryosections. However, due to the highly acid nature of the stain and to the use of a dye with an ionic weight of 763, the method is not applicable to glycol-methacrylate sections (see Gerrits et al 1990). There are no restrictions in terms of fixative used.

➤ Is this procedure easy to carry out?

This method is simple and the inexperienced worker can expect good results.

➤ Obtaining and keeping reliable reagents

1. Fast Green is typically of high and uniform dye content (Wilson 1979). Its most common substitute, Light Green, is more prone to fading.

2. The staining solution is stable for several weeks at room temperature.

➤ Useful routine control procedures

1. To check that a batch of stain is not overaged, stain a section from a specimen known to give good results, as a reagent control. When the colour balance shifts to decreased reds and increased violet tones, make up fresh staining solution.

PROBLEMS AND HOW TO DEAL WITH THEM

➤ Tissue stains unexpectedly weakly

1. If the collagen stains pale blue, but without a red tinge, reduce the time in the poststaining acetic acid rinse.

➤ **Staining is of an unexpected color**

1. If the staining has a yellowish tinge, check if you used tissue fixed in Bouin's fluid. If so, wash the hydrated sections in running tap water to remove residual picric acid.

2. The color balance is altered by dye-bath acidity. If the staining is too red check that the apparent pH is 2 or below. If necessary, adjust downwards using 0.1 M hydrochloric acid.

3. The color balance is affected by prolonged staining times, so do not leave the sections in the Coplin jar over a prolonged period.

4. The color balance is altered by dye ratios, so try adjusting the dye ratio.

➤ **Nature of staining is unusual**

1. Certain pathologically altered collagen (e.g. in burns) may stain red not blue.

2. If fine collagen fibers, or basal laminae, appear fuzzy, try increasing the acidity of the dye-bath by adding 1% concentrated hydrochloric acid.

Background reading

For the original method, with comments on possible substitute dyes, see Gomori (1950). The debated modes of action of systems containing dyes of different sizes plus a heteropoly acid have been reviewed by Kiernan (1990: 121).

18 Gordon and Sweet's stain for reticulin

Background information

This is a silver stain, the metal-impregnation step of which is carried out with a strongly alkaline aqueous solution of a silver ammine. Crucial staining steps are: oxidation with permanganate; mordanting with iron alum; silver impregnation; reduction with formalin; and, if required, gold toning.

The staining mechanism is complex. An initial oxidation generates aldehyde (i.e. reducing) groups in polysaccharide-rich structures in the specimen, including certain collagen fibers ('reticulin'). Exposure to an alkaline silver ammine solution results in two distinct types of silver uptake. First, a loose nonspecific binding of silver cations occurs at most tissue sites. Second, formation of microcrystals of metallic silver, due to reduction of silver cations by aldehyde-rich structures. Subsequently, these microcrystals act as catalytic sites where silver cations, diffusing from surrounding tissues, are reduced by formalin to generate larger crystals of metallic silver, which are responsible for the visible staining. The gold toning deposits gold at the site of the silver, again catalyzed by the silver crystals.

Due to this complexity many factors can, and often do, influence staining. Sensitivity requires retention of polysaccharide in the fibers. This is probably the reason why non-aqueous fixatives often give darker staining than do aqueous ones, as they will retain more polysaccharide. Sensitivity is also increased by rises in temperature or in the concentration of silver ions or in the pH of the solution. However, selectivity is also pH dependent, via site-selective effects in the formation of silver microcrystals. The optimum alkalinity for reticulin staining is above pH 11, and lower than that for other tissue elements.

See Plate 10.

Common variants

Standard staining manuals agree on a single procedure for the Gordon and Sweet stain. However, there are a number of similar silver stains, such as Gomori's and Wilder's stains.

AVOIDING PROBLEMS

➤ **What types of specimen processing are suitable?**

The method can be applied to both paraffin sections and cryosections. Sections cut from hydrophilic resin blocks have also been used, although section swelling and wrinkling in the strongly alkaline impregnation solution may occur in this case.

➤ **Is this procedure easy to carry out?**

As indicated above, opportunities for error are numerous, not least when preparing the impregnation solution. However, with the help of an experienced mentor, the procedure can be considered routine.

➤ **Obtaining and keeping a reliable reagent**

1. Preparation of the silver impregnation reagent is tricky. If inexperienced, seek a mentor. If such a person is not available, seek detailed written advice, perhaps the most explicit being that offered by Gallyas (1979).

2. Store the impregnation reagent in a dark bottle. The use

of a plastic rather than glass bottle has been recommended on safety grounds, since dry silver ammines are unstable to the point of hazard.

PROBLEMS AND HOW TO DEAL WITH THEM

➤ Stain or staining solution not as expected

1. The silver impregnation solution may contain either excess or insufficient ammonia. Carry out solution preparation with care and, if possible, ask the advice of an experienced worker.

2. Ammonia is constantly lost from the impregnation solution by evaporation, eventually giving unstable solutions with poor staining properties. Avoid methods that do not use ammonia in excess. Stain in a Coplin jar to reduce evaporation.

➤ Tissue stains unexpectedly weakly

1. The polysaccharide, which gives rise to the staining, is water soluble and can be lost prior to silver reduction. If unfixed cryosections were used, try fixing them prior to staining; if an aqueous fixative was used, try a nonaqueous one; if a microwave-accelerated variant was used, try reducing preimpregnation temperatures.

2. To increase staining intensities, try increasing the silver concentration or the temperature of the impregnation step. (*Beware*: High background staining may result).

3. Hydrophobic resin embedding media, such as the epoxies using for electron microscopy, can fail to stain, due to exclusion of hydrophilic staining reagents (Horobin 1983). Try removing the resin with an etching agent prior to staining.

➤ Unexpected structures stain

1. Nonselective staining of other tissue elements can occur

if the alkalinity of the silver impregnation solution falls below pH 11. Check that ammonia is not lost.

2. If cell nuclei stain overintensely, try reducing the time in the alum mordant solution.

3. When hydrophilic resin embedding media are used, silver can be retained in the embedding medium, resulting in strong background staining. This is sometimes pronounced when using microwave-accelerated variants. Try extending the preincubation rinse; but beware that too much silver is not lost, so reducing sensitivity.

Background reading

The most extensive scientific investigations of silver staining, including that involved in the Gordon and Sweet procedure, are those by Gallyas (see, in particular, Gallyas 1979, 1982). Other useful studies include a critical account by Puchtler & Sweat Waldrop (1978), and the impressive earlier work of Peters (1955a,b).

Individual staining procedures

19 Gram stain for bacteria, including Gram–Twort and other variants

Background information

The routine procedure uses two cationic dyes, one blue and one red. The blue stain is Crystal Violet, a slightly hydrophobic compound easily precipitated from aqueous solution by hydrophobic anions. The precipitate dissolves in organic solvents having high dielectric constants. The secondary basic dye is most commonly Basic Fuchsin, Neutral Red or Safranin. When staining bacteria in tissue sections, an acid dye counterstain may also be used; with the Gram–Twort stain this is Fast Green; with the Brown and Brenn methods it is picric acid. The routine Gram stain uses tri-iodide anion (present in Gram's iodine) as a hydrophobic anion. The differentiating solvent is most commonly acetone or ethanol ('alcohol'), although aniline–xylene is still recommended in some circumstances.

The routine Gram stain involves an initial Crystal Violet treatment, resulting in coloration of all types of bacteria and, when present, other cells and tissue materials. Treatment with iodine follows, and a subsequent differentiation in acetone or alcohol results in the removal of most Crystal Violet from background material and from some (Gram-negative) organisms. Treatment with the red dye counterstains Gram-negative organisms. Certain variants used with tissue sections, such as the Gram–Twort, use both the basic dye and an acid dye in the counterstaining step.

Initial uptake of microorganisms by Crystal Violet is by basic dyeing of anionic DNA and ribosomal RNA by the cationic dye. Selectivity is provided by the rate-controlled loss of the dye into the differentiator: any factor slowing dye loss can give rise to Gram positivity. For instance, Gram-positive bacteria have much thicker cell walls than do Gram-negative species. In keeping with this, mycobacteria, which have extremely thick cell walls, are Gram positive even if the iodine treatment is not used; Gram-positive organisms become Gram negative following gross structural damage; and Gram-positive substances in animal tissues include such dense (and so impermeable) entities as secretion granules and keratin.

The function of the 'iodine' treatment preceding the differentiation step is to convert the Crystal Violet into a tri-iodide salt of low solubility; this slows the differentiation process down to the point where it is technically practicable.

The counterstain in the routine methods is another cationic dye, which replaces the last traces of Crystal Violet in the permeable Gram-negative organisms, binding to the anionic nucleic acids, and may partially stain the Gram-positive organisms. In the Gram–Twort procedure, the presence of Fast Green in the counterstain and the use of acidic differentiators means that the protein of background cells is stained by acid dyeing; the same applies to the picric acid staining in Brown and Brenn methods.

See Plate 11.

Common variants

As noted above, either Basic Fuchsin, Neutral Red or Safranin are suitable counterstains in routine methods. Substitutes for 'iodine' have included compounds containing such hydrophobic anions as picrate. A variety of differentiators have been used, as noted above.

Among the widely used variants is the Gram–Twort, which

is used for tissue sections, the background being stained with Fast Green.

AVOIDING PROBLEMS

➤ What types of specimen processing are suitable?

The Gram method does not seem particularly fixative sensitive, although heat overfixation can occur. In histopathology, it is routinely carried out on formalin-fixed paraffin sections.

➤ Is this procedure easy to carry out?

These methods are tricky, due to the repeated differentiation and 'wash' steps. Some variants, such as the Gram–Twort and its analogues, are also rather complicated.

The inexperienced will find various options increase the consistency of organism differentiation:

(a) Use of wet fixation rather than using heat;

(b) using a solution of high iodine content, such as Burke's rather than the traditional Gram's;

(c) using a 'slow' differentiator such as propanol rather than acetone or acetic acid variants.

Since there are so many aspects of this procedure that can give trouble, a set routine is recommended even for the experienced worker.

➤ Obtaining and keeping reliable reagents

1. High dye content commercial materials, which more readily differentiate Gram-positive and Gram-negative organisms, are available for Crystal Violet, Neutral Red and Safranin. Purchasing Biological Stain Commission certified samples is the simplest way of achieving this.

2. Although all three of the above dyes can contain minor impurities, there is no indication of this leading to staining errors.

3. Much the same comments apply to the Fast Green used in the Gram–Twort method.

4. Note that different cosolutes (e.g. aniline, phenol and ammonium oxalate) may be added to the Crystal Violet solution. (*Beware:* Such additives can have marked effects on the stability of the dye solution.)

➤ **Useful routine control procedures**

1. Retain samples showing Gram-positive and Gram-negative organisms and use these as positive controls.

PROBLEMS AND HOW TO DEAL WITH THEM

➤ **Tissue stains unexpectedly weakly**

1. If both Gram-positive and Gram-negative controls appear well stained, but the organisms are pale in the specimen being investigated, check that the specimen has not been exposed to acid media, such as fixatives or decalcifying fluids, as these can extract DNA and RNA and so reduce basophilia.

2. If bacterial smears are heat fixed, exposure to a humid atmosphere prior to staining increases the subsequent rate of differentiation, so that Gram-positive organisms may appear Gram negative. If you suspect this is happening, take from heat fixing straight into the staining solution or, alternatively, wet fix the smears in 95% alcohol, since such maneuvers reduce such effects.

3. It is possible to remove all the Crystal Violet by an overextended water wash following the primary staining. Do not go for coffee!

4. If specimens are taken into the differentiator when still wet, then de-colorization can be many times faster, leading to dye loss and thus an apparent lack of Gram-positive organisms. Standardize your procedure: always introduce specimens either wet or dry.

5. In any event, differentiators vary greatly in their tenden-

cy to remove primary dye. If you have trouble of this kind when using acetone or ethanol differentiators, reduce the amount of water in the differentiator, or try alternative differentiators, such as propanol or aniline xylene (the latter, however, is more toxic).

6. Note that the Gram–Twort variant, which uses acetic acid–alcohol for short periods as differentiator, is particularly prone to overdifferentiation. Ensure the slide is completely dry before differentiation, as the presence of such carried-over water increases the speed of differentiation.

7. If the counterstain seems too pale, check, and perhaps reduce, the length of the poststaining water washing and also note the previous comment.

➤ Unexpected structures stain

1. If specimens are allowed to dry before being taken into the differentiator, then de-colorization can be many times slower, leading to an apparent excess of Gram-positive organisms. Standardize your procedure: always introduce specimens either wet or dry and adjust the differentiation time appropriately.

2. Nonbacterial Gram-positive material that may appear in smears includes some fungi. In tissue sections, elastin, fibrin, keratin, and Paneth cell and other secretion granules may also be Gram-positive.

3. Gram-positive particles of varying sizes and shapes can appear in urine sediments. If the specimen was heat fixed, these may be damaged bacteria, so try chemically fixing such specimens (see Hyman 1992). If such material appears in chemically fixed sediments, consider if it could derive from the lubricant used for catheterization.

➤ Nature of staining is unusual

1. If the differential staining of Gram-positive and Gram-negative organisms is poor, check the thickness of the

preparation. In this rate-controlled procedure, specimen thickness influences dye diffusion, and hence thin preparations are called for.

► **Other problems**

1. Inconsistent staining can occur with tissue sections following acid decalcification of the block. Use EDTA decalcifiers if proposing to stain by Gram methods.

Background reading

This method attracts comments such as 'its chemical rationale is still obscure' and 'the mechanism of action remains unknown'. This is particularly ironic, since in the early 1950s Bartholamew and his collaborators defined the mechanism of the Gram stain with a precision rarely seen with other standard staining methods (Mittwer et al 1950, Bartholamew & Mittwer 1950, 1951). Later, this group also clarified the causes of many staining problems and set out a rational standardized Gram procedure for smears (Bartholamew 1962, Tucker & Bartholamew 1962). For a brief description of this work, see Horobin (1988: 80).

For reviews of Gram staining set in a modern context, see Popescu & Doyle (1996) and Scherrer (1984). It is of interest that the first of these reviews essentially agrees with the rationale favored by the present authors, and cites the papers of Bartholamew, and yet does not see them as key.

20 Grimelius' silver method for argyrophil cells

Background information

This is an argyrophil silver method, so it stains materials that can be impregnated with silver, but that require a reducing agent to produce the black derivative of metallic silver. The metal impregnation step is in silver nitrate; reduction is by hydroquinone; and counterstaining uses any suitable dye (e.g. Neutral Red).

Crucial staining steps are: silver impregnation carried out with a hot, slightly acidic, aqueous solution of silver nitrate; reduction in a warm aqueous solution of hydroquinone; and, if required, counterstaining.

The silver staining process involves two key steps. During exposure to the silver nitrate some metal cations become loosely bound to a wide variety of tissue sites; in addition, microcrystals of metallic silver are formed due to reduction of silver cations by the biogenic amines of the argyrophil cells. Subsequently, these microcrystals act as catalytic sites where silver cations, diffusing from surrounding structures, are reduced by the hydroquinone to generate more and larger crystals of metallic silver, which are responsible for the visible staining. Counterstaining can utilize acid or basic dyeing, to provide background coloration.

See Plate 12.

AVOIDING PROBLEMS

➤ **What types of specimen processing are suitable?**

The method is routinely applied to Bouin-fixed paraffin sections. Although formalin can also be used, it gives less intense staining.

➤ **Is this procedure easy to carry out?**

The only awkward step is the use of microscopic control to ensure that staining remains selective whilst becoming intense.

➤ **Obtaining and keeping reliable reagents**

1. The working solutions should be freshly prepared.

PROBLEMS AND HOW TO DEAL WITH THEM

➤ **Tissue stains unexpectedly weakly**

1. As the stain ages, coloration becomes less intense, so check whether you used freshly prepared solutions.

2. To increase staining intensities, return the section to the impregnation bath for a short period. (*Guideline*: Try 5 min in the first instance.)

Background reading

For the original account of this stain, see Grimelius (1968). The most extensive scientific investigations of silver staining are those by Gallyas (see, in particular, Gallyas 1979, 1982).

21 Grocott hexamine (methamine) silver for fungi

Background information

This is a silver stain, the metal impregnation step of which is carried out with a strongly alkaline aqueous solution of silver hexamethamine, a metal coordination complex. Gold chloride is used as an intensifier. A variety of dyes (e.g. the acid dye Light Green) may be used as counterstains.

Crucial staining steps are: oxidation with acidic dichromate, followed by washing in sodium metabisulfite; silver impregnation in warm silver hexamine; intensification with gold chloride; and counterstaining with an acid dye or equivalent.

The initial oxidation generates aldehyde groups in polysaccharide-rich structures in the specimen, including the fungal cell walls. These groups then reduce silver ions present in the alkaline silver ammine solution to metallic silver microcrystals. Subsequent gold toning deposits gold at the site of this silver, the process being catalyzed by the silver crystals themselves. Counterstains vary, but Light Green is applied at low pH, and so gives coloration of tissue proteins by acid dyeing.

See Plate 13.

Common variants

A number of minor variants are to be found in staining manuals. In addition, there are clearly related techniques, such as Gordon and Sweet's and Wilder's. A wide variety of counterstains may be recommended, e.g. the acid dyes Light Green or Fast Green, hematoxylin and Eosin, or various trichromes, such as Arzacs.

AVOIDING PROBLEMS

➤ What types of specimen processing are suitable?

Various fixatives can be used. Bouin's fluid or other formalin-based fixatives result in more effective impregnation. This procedure is routinely carried out on paraffin sections, although sections of tissues in hydrophilic resins such as glycolmethacrylate may also be used; staining of frozen sections is less successful.

➤ Is this procedure easy to carry out?

This is a slow, complicated method, with many opportunities for error; not least the use of microscopic control.

➤ Obtaining and keeping reliable reagents

1. Keep the silver methenamine solution in the refrigerator, where it will be stable for a month or two.

2. Prepare the working solution of the silver impregnation system immediately prior to use, as it is unstable.

3. Store the impregnation reagent in a dark bottle. The use of a plastic rather than glass bottle has been recommended on safety grounds, since dry silver ammines are unstable to the point of hazard.

➤ Useful routine control procedures

1. Retain a specimen containing fungi, and stain a section from this as a positive control along with the experimental sections.

PROBLEMS AND HOW TO DEAL WITH THEM

➤ **Tissue stains unexpectedly weakly**

1. Use positive controls known to contain fungi, to check that staining solutions have not deteriorated. If necessary, prepare fresh solutions.

2. Incubation times required vary with fixative and duration of fixation. Use microscopic control, aiming for dark-brown fungi with a colorless background. (*Guideline*: Try incubating for 60 mins in the first instance.)

➤ **Unexpected structures stain**

1. This method is not specific for fungi, and other polysaccharide-containing materials (e.g. chitin, glycogen, mucins and starch) will stain. Materials able to reduce silver cations without prior oxidation, such as melanin, will also stain. Deposits of insoluble calcium salts may also blacken, especially if light is not excluded.

2. If connective tissue elements stain, reduce the incubation time.

3. If background remains, even after reducing incubation times, check that the impregnation was carried out in the dark.

4. If random deposits of stain occur (e.g. on the glassware) ensure you use chemically clean glassware and avoid contact with metal items (e.g. use plastic forceps for handling impregnated slides), as such contamination can reduce silver cations directly or by acting as catalysts.

5. Moreover, check that the Coplin jar is sealed during the impregnation and that the temperature of the oven or water bath does not go above 60°C, as the silver ammine complex is unstable at higher temperatures.

➤ **Nature of staining is unusual**

1. If the staining of fungi is so intense that details of the

hyphal septae are obscured, reduce the incubation time. Identification of fungi requires this detail, and is best seen in underimpregnated sections.

➤ Other problems

1. If the sections lift off the slides, check that the temperature is not above 60°C, and that the lid of the Coplin jar is well fitting. Some workers celloidinize their sections, but if you do this it may be necessary to remove strongly stained celloidin with acetone during dehydration.

Background reading

The method described here was originally derived by Grocott (1955) from one previously described by Gomori. The most extensive scientific investigations of silver staining are those of Gallyas (see, in particular, Gallyas 1979, 1982).

22 Hematoxylin and Eosin as an oversight stain

Background information

In this entry, as in the routine laboratory, 'hematoxylin' is shorthand for aluminum hematoxylin. Eosin is routinely Eosin Y.

Regarding aluminum hematoxylin, there are many variants. However, they all probably contain, or give rise to, hydrophilic cationic complexes of hematin and aluminum. The hematin arises from oxidation of hematoxylin; a source of aluminum ions then being added. Eosin Y is an acid dye, with a slightly lipophilic colored anion of moderate size.

There are even more hematoxylin and Eosin staining procedures than hematoxylins, and a generic procedure follows. Sections are first stained in a hematoxylin solution. Progressive stains continue this until the desired intensity is achieved. Regressive stains are overstained at this point. Specimens are next treated with dilute alkali (tap water, in some towns) until the reddish staining is transformed to a blue-black form (bluing). A wash in acid alcohol follows. This is either a brief rinse to remove unbound stain (for progressive staining), or is a differentiation, often under microscopic control (for regressive staining). Sections are then re-blued if necessary. Sections are counterstained in Eosin Y.

Such hematoxylin and Eosin staining comprises basic dyeing followed by acid dying. The cationic metal-complex dye stains anionic biopolymers (DNA, RNA and glycosaminoglycans), and the anionic dye stains cationic proteins. Unlike many basic dyes, hematoxylin is not lost into dehydration fluids, as its hydrophilicity reduces alcohol solubility. However, the acidic differentiator breaks the complex, releasing hematin, which is readily lost. Other peculiarities of hematoxylin staining (e.g. some variants stain glycosaminoglycans, and others elastic fibers, and some neither) may be attributed to the variable salt content of the different staining solutions.

Despite its complications, hematoxylin and Eosin staining is robust, hence the method's long-term use. Thus, neither hematoxylin nor Eosin staining are sensitive to the mode of fixation. Intensity of hematoxylin staining depends on the times of staining and of differentiation; selectivity is most influenced by the amount of electrolyte present, this property varying from one type of hematoxylin to another.

Common variants

There are many hematoxylins, and widely used examples are reviewed by Stevens & Wilson (1996). In summary, the amount of hematoxylin, the amount of nonaqueous solvents and acids, the amount of oxidant, the times and temperatures of the oxidation, and the amount and type of aluminum salt may all vary in different procedures.

Hematoxylins such as Ehrlich's and Delafield's, prepared using atmospheric oxygen, are termed 'naturally ripened'. Hematoxylins such as Harris' or Mayer's, prepared using oxidants such as mercuric oxide or sodium iodate, are termed 'chemically ripened'.

Variants often carry the names of the workers who devised a particular formulation, as above. Carzzi's and Cole's hematoxylins are other currently recommended variants.

Freshly prepared hematoxylins may contain the aluminum–dye complex plus varying amounts of hematin, free aluminum ions, and free hematoxylin (e.g. Ehrlich's or

Individual staining procedures

Delafield's). Note that the composition often changes as the solution ages. 'Aluminum hematoxylin' is neither a single nor a standardized stain.

AVOIDING PROBLEMS

➤ What types of specimen processing are suitable?

Both paraffin and cryosections can be stained satisfactorily, by choosing appropriate staining or differentiation times. Celloidin and resin sections can also be stained, after suitable modifications. Thus, with celloidin sections, absolute ethanol must be avoided and dehydration carried out in butanol. When staining sections of hydrophilic resins, swelling and wrinkling may occur. However, this may be avoided by using suitably formulated resins (see Gerrits & Van Leeuwen 1987).

➤ Is this procedure easy to carry out?

The hematoxylin methods often utilize differentiation, and use microscopic control. Moreover, the stain itself changes as it ages. However, hematoxylins have two major advantages over basic dyes such as Methylene Blue or Crystal Violet. First, differentiation of hematoxylins is slow and easily controlled; and, secondly, inadvertent loss of stain into alcoholic dehydrating fluids does not occur.

➤ Obtaining and keeping reliable reagents

1. Commercial samples of both Eosin and hematoxylin (the metal-free precursor is being referred to here) are usually of high dye content, and low in contaminants.

2. Naturally ripened hematoxylins typically require 2–4 months to ripen. However, chemically ripened hematoxylins may be prepared very rapidly.

3. Bulk solutions of naturally ripened hematoxylins retain their staining properties for years. Even in a Coplin jar, activity is usually retained for months. However, even bulk solutions of hematoxylins prepared by chemical

oxidants have shorter shelf-lives of up to 6 months or so.

PROBLEMS AND HOW TO DEAL WITH THEM

▶ Stain or staining solution not as expected

1. The formation of precipitates in chemically ripened hematoxylins indicates deterioration. Filter before use and, if necessary, extend the staining times. If large numbers of slides are stained, prepare a fresh batch of stain each month.

▶ Tissue stains unexpectedly weakly

Hematoxylin staining:

1. If the stain was naturally ripened, check that it has ripened for a sufficient period. The ripening may be speeded up by placing an unstoppered bottle in a warm sunny place. (*Note*: This is being written in the North of England.)

2. If stain was chemically ripened, was the solution prepared several months ago? Or has a precipitate formed in the stock solution? In either case, see 'Stain or staining solution not as expected', above.

3. If stain is heavily used, it will deteriorate more rapidly. Try longer staining times.

4. Specimens exposed to acidic solutions prior to staining (e.g. decalcification media, or unbuffered formalin or picric acid fixatives) may lose DNA and hence require longer staining times.

5. If hematoxylin-stained sections are exposed to acidic solutions, such as Van Gieson's stain, the stain decomposes. In such cases use an alternative stain, such as an iron hematoxylin, or an iron Celestine Blue method.

6. Tissues embedded in hydrophilic resins may stain slowly due to occlusion (Gerrits et al 1991). Lengthen staining times, or add a little alcohol to the stain.

➤ Unexpected structures stain

1. Overstaining with hematoxylin can occur under various circumstances:

    (a) If the standard protocols, typically designed for paraffin sections, are applied unmodified to frozen sections or cytological specimens. Reduce the staining times appreciably; in the first instance, try halving them.

    (b) If tissues are embedded in hydrophilic resin, high resin background staining can occur (Gerrits et al 1991). Try differentiating in alcohol.

2. Overstaining with Eosin can occur with routine procedures if mercuric fixations have been used. Shorten the Eosin staining time, or lengthen the poststaining wash.

➤ Staining is of an unexpected color

1. Yellowish or brownish tinges seen following hematoxylin staining may be due to the stain being contaminated with oxyhematin (Marshal & Horobin 1972). If this is a problem, prepare a fresh batch of stain.

➤ Other problems

1. If tissue is embedded in a water-miscible resin, such as glycolmethacrylate, and the resin wrinkles after hematoxylin staining, try modifying the resin following the suggestions of Gerrits & Van Leeuwen (1987).

Background reading

A useful overview of hematoxylin and Eosin stains is available (Stevens & Wilson 1996), as is a brief account of the mechanism of hematoxylin and Eosin staining (Horobin 1988). Note that the latter account disputes the traditional mechanistic viewpoint on hematoxylin staining, namely that it involves mordanting (i.e. the formation of metal ion–tissue covalent bonds). For an account of the latter, see Baker (1962).

A discussion of the role of salt on staining patterns seen with hematoxylins is given in Marshall & Horobin (1973). A more recent investigation of hematoxylin staining by Bettinger & Zimmermann (1991) indicates that neither mordanting nor large conjugated systems are significant. This work also establishes the structures of the aluminum–hematin complexes on a sound chemical footing.

23 Jones's hexamine silver method for basement membranes and basal laminae

Background information

This is a silver stain in which metal impregnation is carried out with a strongly alkaline aqueous solution of a silver ammine. Intensification uses gold chloride; counterstaining may use a variety of acid and basic dyes.

Crucial staining steps are: oxidation with periodate; silver impregnation with hot, aqueous silver methenamine; and, if required, gold toning.

The initial periodate oxidation generates aldehyde (i.e. reducing) groups selectively in polysaccharide-rich structures in the specimen. Exposure to an alkaline silver ammine solution results in the formation of microcrystals of metallic silver, due to reduction of silver cations by aldehydes.

The subsequent gold toning deposits gold at the site of the silver crystals, this process being catalyzed by the silver crystals themselves. Typical counterstains are Light Green or hematoxylin and Eosin; for the staining mechanisms of these stains, see the Index.

See Plate 14.

Common variants

Jones's variant was modified from the original of Gomori

(1946). As well as Gomori's stain, the Gordon and Sweet's and Wilder's stains have obvious similarities.

AVOIDING PROBLEMS

➤ What types of specimen preparation are suitable?

Routinely, Bouin's fluid is used for fixation; formalin is satisfactory but requires longer impregnation times; and heavy metal containing fixatives should be avoided.

The method can be applied both to paraffin and cryosections. Sections cut from hydrophilic resin blocks have also been used, although further problems may arise in this case; including section swelling and wrinkling in the strongly alkaline impregnation solution.

➤ Is this procedure easy to carry out?

This is a somewhat laborious method, not least when preparing the impregnation solution and when achieving selective staining under microscopic control. However, the procedure does demonstrate the finer basement membranes, such as those of the glomerulus, very well indeed.

➤ Obtaining and keeping reliable reagents

1. Store the impregnation reagent in a dark bottle in the refrigerator. A plastic rather than glass bottle has been recommended on safety grounds, since dry silver ammines are unstable to the point of hazard. Under these conditions solutions will be stable for several weeks.

PROBLEMS AND HOW TO DEAL WITH THEM

➤ Tissue stains unexpectedly weakly

1. To increase staining intensities, try extending the time of the silver impregnation. (*Guideline*: Start at 20 min, if the temperature of the impregnation bath is 56°C.)

➤ Unexpected structures stain

1. If granular background deposits occur, check if a heavy metal fixative was used. Such fixatives should be avoided.

➤ Other problems

If excessive wrinkling or swelling of glycolmethacrylate resin sections occurs, try increasing the amount of cross-linker used in the resin formulation, slightly.

Background reading

For the original Jones method, see Jones (1957). The most extensive scientific investigations of silver staining are those by Gallyas (see Gallyas 1979, 1982). Other useful studies include a critical account by Puchtler & Sweat Waldrop (1978), and the impressive earlier work by Peters (1955a,b).

Individual staining procedures

24 Lactase by an indigogenic method

Background information

This method requires a substrate, in the form of an indoxyl derivative, and an oxidant, comprising a mixture of ferro- and ferricyanide ions. The substrate is the 5-bromo-4-chloroindoxyl-β-D-fucoside or -fucopyranoside; the halogenation of the indolyl ring increases substantivity and decreases water solubility.

Selectivity is achieved by use of the tailored substrates. These substrates are converted by lactase into colorless intermediate reaction products, indoxyls, which condense to form indigo dyes. The oxidative condensation is accelerated by the ferro-/ferricyanide oxidant. Localization at the enzymic site is favored by the low solubility of the halogenated substrate.

AVOIDING PROBLEMS

➤ **What types of specimen processing are suitable?**

Unfixed cryostat sections; or, if fixed, use only cold formol preferably with a colloid protecting agent.

➤ **Is this procedure easy to carry out?**

The procedure is straightforward, but slow. As the substrate is poorly soluble, it must be brought into solution in an organic solvent such as dimethylformamide before mixing with other constituents. The final indigo dye is extremely substantive, so the sections can be mounted in any medium without problems.

➤ Obtaining and keeping reliable reagents

1. If the medium is to be re-used (and the substrate is expensive) then it must be filtered and stored frozen at −20°C between uses. If this is done the incubation medium can be re-used up to ten times with typical specimens.

PROBLEMS AND HOW TO DEAL WITH THEM

➤ Tissue stains unexpectedly weakly

1. Lactase is inhibited by formaldehyde, so postfix in formalin following incubation.

➤ Unexpected structures stain

1. If the staining appears diffuse, try shorter incubation times.

Background reading

The method is described in Lojda et al (1979) and in Filipe & Lake (1990).

25 Leucine aminopeptidase for demonstration of proteases

Background information

This simultaneous coupling procedure uses two key reagents: a synthetic organic naphthylamide as substrate, and a diazonium salt as visualizing agent. The use of copper ions to immobilize the final reaction product may be carried out with certain diazonium salts.

Routinely, the substrate is L-leucyl-4-methoxy-β-naphthylamide, or L-leucyl-β-naphthylamide. These compounds do not have extended conjugated systems, unlike the AS naphthols. The usual diazonium salt used is Fast Blue B.

This is a simultaneous-coupling azodye procedure, so the substrate and visualizing agent are applied together. Selectivity is achieved by substrate specificity.

During incubation the enzyme converts the naphthylamide to naphthylamine, which couples with the diazonium salt to yielding an azodye. This colored derivative is often subsequently converted into a 2 : 1 dye/copper chelate. This metal complex has a conjugated system twice the size of the parent dye. Consequently, van der Waals attractions are favored, and the metal complex binds tightly to tissue proteins. This provides good localization, and resistance to extraction by mountants.

See Plate 15.

Common variants

The routine substrate is L-leucyl-4-methoxy-β-naphthylamide, but L-leucyl-β-naphthylamide can also be used. Other fast salts have been used as visualizing agents (e.g. Fast Black K, Fast Garnet G, and Fast Red B). However, use of the postincubation copper chelation step to improve stain localization requires the diazonium salt to be Fast Blue B. If this latter variant is carried out, mounting may be in any medium, including the technically superior resins.

AVOIDING PROBLEMS

> ➤ **What types of specimen processing are suitable?**

The successful use of a variety of fixative and specimen-preparation methods has been reported, including cell smears, but cryostat sections prefixed in formalin are often used.

> ➤ **Is this procedure easy to carry out?**

The procedure is straightforward.

> ➤ **Obtaining and keeping reliable reagents**

1. Commercial diazonium (i.e. 'fast') salts contain stabilizer, and can be stored long-term in the refrigerator. However, prepare solutions freshly for each stain, since once dissolved the salts deteriorate.

> ➤ **Useful routine control procedures**

1. Positive controls are essential with this method.
2. Also, omit the substrate in order to check that staining is enzymic in origin.

PROBLEMS AND HOW TO DEAL WITH THEM

> ➤ **Tissue stains unexpectedly weakly**

1. As fixation can inhibit the enzyme, try using unfixed

cryosections, especially if the tissue under study is expected to have a low enzyme content.

2. Optimum incubation times and temperatures depend on the activity of the particular tissue under study, so try longer incubation times or higher incubation temperatures.

3. Optimum incubation pH for arylamidases demonstrated histochemically is usually in the range 5.5–6.8, so check the pH of your incubation medium, and adjust it downwards if necessary.

4. One report suggests that Tris buffer inhibits arylamidases: avoid this buffer.

5. Some diazonium salts, including Fast Blue RR, are unstable in solution. Make sure the fast salt is dissolved immediately prior to incubating the slide. Indeed, if the incubation is prolonged, replace the incubation medium as staining proceeds.

6. The stabilizers present in certain batches of fast salts, or the fast salts themselves, are enzyme inhibitory. So try another batch of fast salt, from a different source, preferably one stated to be stabilized by a different counter ion; or try a different fast salt.

7. Decomposition of the diazonium salts increases as the temperature is raised, so check this if you incubated above room temperature.

8. Several reasons have been suggested as to why cyanide ions enhance staining (e.g. enzyme activation, and chelation of inhibiting inorganic ions), so check that cyanide ion was present.

➤ **Unexpected structures stain**

1. If diffuse staining occurs around the enzymic site, check if prestaining fixation was used, and if not try such fixation.

2. In any case, check if a postincubation copper chelation procedure was used, and if not try this.

3. The degree of stain diffusion also depends on the diazonium salt used, so use Fast Blue B, if you are not doing so already.

4. The degree of stain diffusion also depends on the substrate, so check that you were not using L-leucyl-β-naphthylamide, since this gives a less substantive reaction product.

5. Staining of lipids or lipid-rich materials can occur when hydrophobic naphthols are used. In such circumstances, make sure you use the postincubation copper chelation step, as the chelate is not likely to exhibit this artifact. Alternatively, extract the section with a lipid solvent (e.g. hot chloroform–methanol) prior to staining. Since this staining is nonenzymic, it will also be detected by routine control procedure 2 (see above).

6. Yellowish-brown background staining can arise when Fast Red RR is used, due to the reaction of this diazonium salt with tissue proteins. If such a background goes reddish blue with the copper after treatment, and not bright blue, ignore it.

7. There are species differences in enzyme distribution. Make sure you know what to expect in your specimen.

8. After specimens stained with the copper-chelated Fast Blue RR derived azodye have been stored for some months, nuclear staining can occur. So check the age of your preparation.

➤ Nature of staining is unusual

1. Gross crystallization of the azodye, obscuring cellular detail, can arise, especially with certain substrates and fast salts, and if the copper chelation step is not used. Use the methoxy substituted substrate, Fast Blue RR, and copper after-treatment.

Background reading

The copper chelate variant of this procedure is described in some detail and its mode of action discussed in a paper from Seligman's group (Nachlas et al 1957). Another useful review of arylamidase histochemistry may be found in Chayen & Bitensky (1991: 188–190). Pathological applications can be found in Filipe & Lake (1990).

26 Luxol Fast Blue for myelin

Background information

Luxol Fast Blue MBS was the dye originally used for this procedure. However, Luxol Fast Blue A and G have also been used. These are all acid dyes, probably with large conjugated systems and hydrophilic anions. Unusually, their counter-ions are hydrophobic organic cations. Consequently, the dyes are insoluble in water and hydrocarbons but soluble in polar organic solvents. Differences between the three dyes noted above exist, but are small. Hence in this entry the dyes are not distinguished, and are referred to generically as Luxol Fast Blue.

The use of Luxol Fast Blue to stain myelin requires an initial prolonged treatment with dye dissolved in hot, slightly acidic ethanol or methanol. This colors myelin, but not other lipids, and in addition gives a general background staining of acidophilic materials. The latter is removed by differentiating alternately in aqueous alkali and aqueous alcohol. Note that elastic fibers, eosinophil granules and erythrocytes remain colored after this differentiation.

Uptake of Luxol Fast Blue into phospholipid-rich structures is a consequence of the hydrophobic cations and of the use of nonaqueous solvents. Under these conditions ion pairing is maximized. The organic cation–dye anion pairs will be lipophilic, and will partition into the hydrophobic myelin. The background staining is acid dyeing of cationic tissue proteins by the dye anions, which also occurs in myelin. Background staining is largely lost during differentiation in aqueous alkali, as proteins will then carry anionic charges. Structures retaining dye are either dense (and thus slow to de-stain), favor van der Waals binding, or are hydrophobic (and so exclude the hydrophilic differentiator). Dye is retained by the myelin, since this material is both hydrophobic and dense.

Consequently, the sensitivity is dependent on the solvent polarity: if too polar, ion pairs will not form; if insufficiently polar, partitioning into lipids is not favored. Selectivity is dependent on differentiation. Prior to differentiation, permeable hydrophilic protein-rich structures such as collagen fibers are well stained. However, dense and/or hydrophobic structures de-stain slowly.

Common variants

Either ethanolic or methanolic dye solutions may be used, the overall polarity being adjusted by suitable amounts of water. Any of the Luxol Fast Blue dyes are satisfactory, although they are not identical.

AVOIDING PROBLEMS

➤ **What types of specimen processing are suitable?**

The procedure may be applied to paraffin and celloidin sections.

➤ **Is this procedure easy to carry out?**

The method is simpler than traditional alternatives, such as the Weigert–Pal hematoxylin procedures. However, it is rather slow, especially with thick neuroanatomical sections.

➤ **Obtaining and keeping reliable reagents**

1. Although several different dyes may be supplied under

the name Luxol Fast Blue, all may be used for this procedure, although they will not give identical results.

2. Acidified methanolic stock solutions of Luxol Fast Blue A have been reported to remain satisfactory for up to 18 months.

PROBLEMS AND HOW TO DEAL WITH THEM

➤ Tissue stains unexpectedly weakly

1. Patchy staining may be due to a failure of fixation, as may some weak coloration. Try extending the fixation time, or using smaller tissue blocks. If formalin fixation has been used, try adding cetylpyridinium bromide to the solution (Salthouse 1962).

2. Weak staining occurs if the solvent becomes too polar. This can occur in various ways, for instance if sections are taken down to water rather than to 95% alcohol. Check the actual procedure used, habits are strong. The amount of water in the ethanol or methanol may also vary, so check this with care.

3. Fine myelinated fibers can be overdifferentiated. If single fibers are being traced, use microscopic control of differentiator.

➤ Unexpected structures stain

1. High background staining (e.g. of collagen fibers) can arise if differentiation is incomplete. Try extending differentiation, perhaps using microscopic control.

2. Background staining is also rather more likely with methanolic than with ethanolic dye-baths. Try an ethanolic variant.

Background reading

An account of the ion-pairing/differentiation mechanism of Luxol Fast Blue staining is available (Clasen et al 1973).

Staining of myelin was originally considered to be due to chemical, rather than biophysical, selectivity (e.g. Lycette et al 1970).

27 Masson–Fontana procedure for melanin and other argentaffin materials

Background information

This is an argentaffin method, that is to say it stains those materials that reduce silver salts in the dark, without the aid of an external reducing agent. The metal impregnation step is carried out with a strongly alkaline aqueous solution of a silver ammine. The intensification reagent is gold chloride. Any appropriate counterstain can be used (e.g. Neutral Red or Safranin).

Crucial staining steps are: silver impregnation in aqueous alkaline silver ammine, by either hot or room temperature methods; optional intensification with gold chloride; and, if required, counterstaining.

During exposure to the alkaline silver ammine solution, the quinone groups of the melanin reduce silver cations, forming deposits of metallic silver. The gold toning precipitates gold at the site of the silver, a process catalyzed by the silver crystals themselves.

See Plate 16.

Common variants

There are room temperature variants with long impregnation times, or quicker 'hot' versions. The former are considered the more precise.

AVOIDING PROBLEMS

➤ **What types of specimen processing are suitable?**

With some adjustments, the method can be applied to paraffin and cryosections, as well as celloidin and resin sections.

➤ **Is this procedure easy to carry out?**

This is a simple method, apart from the preparation of the silver incubation solution.

➤ **Obtaining and keeping reliable reagents**

1. Preparation of the silver impregnation reagent is tricky. If inexperienced, seek a mentor. If such a person is not available, seek detailed written advice, perhaps the most explicit being that offered by Gallyas (1979).

2. Store the impregnation reagent in the refrigerator, in a dark bottle, under which conditions it should be satisfactory for several weeks. Use plastic rather than glass bottles for storage, on safety grounds.

➤ **Useful routine control procedures**

1. Retain a specimen containing melanin, and stain sections from this as positive controls.

PROBLEMS AND HOW TO DEAL WITH THEM

➤ **Stain or staining solution not as expected**

1. Ammonia may be lost from the impregnation solution by evaporation, eventually giving unstable solutions with poor staining properties. Stain in a closed Coplin jar to reduce evaporation.

➤ **Tissue stains unexpectedly weakly**

1. To increase staining intensities, raise the temperature or extend the time of the silver impregnation. (*Beware*: High background staining may result.)

2. Note that neuromelanin stains more slowly than other melanins.

▶ Unexpected structures stain

1. This method is not specific for melanin, and also stains argentaffin and chromaffin granules, and some lipofuscins.

2. If a fine precipitate covers the section, check if you used a heated incubation and, if so, try incubating at room temperature.

3. Another cause of random deposits of black material can be reduction of silver cations due to contaminated glassware or the use of metal forceps. Clean all glassware scrupulously and use plastic forceps when moving slides in and out of the impregnation solution.

▶ Other problems

1. If the slide is covered with silver, clean all glassware carefully before use.

2. If the sections lift from the slide, celloidinize the sections before staining.

Background reading

The most extensive scientific investigations of silver staining are those by Gallyas (see, in particular, Gallyas 1979, 1982).

28 Masson's Trichrome

Background information

There have been several variants of the Masson Trichrome. This entry addresses 'generic Masson' issues arising with the variants in current use.

Nuclei are demonstrated using preformed metal complex stains, such as Weigert's iron hematoxylin or iron Celestine Blue–aluminum hematoxylin. Alternatives for the first acid dyeing step include the following commercially available dyes: Acid Fuchsin, Biebrich Scarlet, Bordeaux Red, Chromotrope 2R and Nitrazine Yellow. These 'cytoplasmic' or 'plasma' stains are mostly smallish anionic dyes of slightly hydrophilic character. Commercially available alternatives for the second acid dyeing step include Aniline Blue, Fast Green, Light Green, Lissamine Green and Methyl Blue. These 'collagen' or 'connective tissue' dyes are anionic, typically of moderate size and extremely hydrophilic character.

A 'generic' Masson's Trichrome procedure is as follows. An optional picric acid pretreatment is followed by staining of the nuclei. The first acid dyeing step follows, using one of the dyes noted above applied from an acidic aqueous solution for a few minutes. Next, the section is treated with an extremely acidic solution of a polyacid (usually phosphotungstic acid) for a few minutes. Then, without washing the section, the second acid dyeing step is carried out. Here one of the dyes noted above is applied from an acidic aqueous solution for a few minutes. Finally, the section is differentiated in aqueous acetic acid.

The Masson Trichrome involves acid and basic dyeing. The cationic metal complex dyes stain the polyanions, DNA and RNA. The anionic dyes stain proteins, which are polycations at the low pH used. The basis of differential staining by different anionic dyes, with collagen fibers selectively stained by the second, is disputed. One view considers the staining patterns as rate controlled. The first dye stains all protein-rich sites. The second dye only stains the most permeable sites, namely collagen fibers. From this viewpoint the role of the polyacids is three-fold: to form insoluble pigments with the cationic nuclear stains; to produce an extremely acidic dye-bath; and to act as selective differentiating agents. Several technical factors are congruent with this mechanism. An alternative theoretical perspective considers that the polyacids play a more complex role, perhaps acting as mordants.

Staining selectivity is fixative dependent. Many fixatives may be used, but if these do not contain mercuric chloride or picric acid a prestaining treatment ('mordanting') with Bouin's fluid, or with saturated picric acid or mercuric chloride, has been recommended. Selectivity is also influenced by dye-bath pH, and duration of staining and washing steps.

Common variants

For examples of alternative dyes and choice of fixatives, see above. Some variants use phosphotungstic acid, others a mixture of phosphotungstic acid and phosphomolybdic acid.

AVOIDING PROBLEMS

➤ **What types of specimen processing are suitable?**

The method can be applied to paraffin or cryosections. If used with tissues embedded in hydrophilic resins, use of larger dyes (e.g. Aniline Blue, Fast Green, Light Green or Methyl Blue) should be avoided, or staining of resin occurs. The smaller connective tissue dye Lissamine Green can be substituted.

Since the stain involves highly acidic solutions, wrinkling of resin occurs unless sufficient cross-linker has been used.

➤ Is this procedure easy to carry out?

The procedure is complicated, and beginners may have difficulty in achieving consistent results. However, staining may be inspected after each step, so detailed control is possible.

➤ Obtaining and keeping reliable reagents

Few difficulties arise from impure commercial dye samples in the Masson procedure, perhaps because the method provides repeated opportunities to adjust the color balance as staining proceeds.

PROBLEMS AND HOW TO DEAL WITH THEM

➤ Tissue stains unexpectedly weakly

1. Weak nuclear staining occurs for many reasons. For suggestions concerning aluminum hematoxylin, see Entry 22, p. 88.

2. Understaining by 'cytoplasmic' dyes can arise for a variety of reasons:

    (a) Many cytoplasmic dyes are removed by overextended water washes, leaving the collagen dye in place, as typical cytoplasmic dyes are smaller, and thus faster diffusing, than typical collagen dyes. Check wash times and try shortening them.

    (b) Many cytoplasmic dyes can also be selectively washed out, leaving the collagen dye behind, by overextended alcoholic dehydration, as typical cytoplasmic dyes are more alcohol soluble than typical collagen dyes. Check the dehydration time and try shortening it.

(c) Uneven staining (e.g. where adjacent muscle fibers have markedly different color intensities) can arise if specimens were formalin fixed. If so, check that a Bouin's or picric acid or mercuric chloride mordant was applied prior to staining.

➤ Unexpected structures stain

1. Background staining of the embedding medium can occur when staining tissues embedded in hydrophilic resins. Acid dyes of moderate size (e.g. Aniline Blue, Fast Green, Light Green and Methyl Blue) stain such resins, and are then difficult to remove (see Gerrits et al 1990). Try a recommended connective tissue stain of smaller size (e.g. Wool Green, also known as Acid Green 50 or Lissamine Green).

➤ Staining is of an unexpected color

1. The color balance is fixative dependent. Fixatives increasing rate of staining (e.g. Carnoy's fluid) tend to produce overstaining by the connective tissue stain, while fixatives decreasing rates of staining (e.g. Zenker's fluid) tend to limit staining by the collagen stain to the connective tissue elements.

2. Changes in color balance can also occur in microwave-accelerated procedures, with a tendency for the collagen dye to overstain in heated dye-baths. Reduce the temperature or staining time of the second acid dyeing step.

Background reading

For an elegant discussion of these methods, written from the perspective of the rate control mechanism, see Baker (1958). A more recent review, mentioning the alternative mechanisms, is available in Bancroft & Stevens (1990: 129).

Individual staining procedures

29 Methyl Green–Pyronin for plasma cells

Background information

Traditional Methyl Green, which contains seven methyl substituents, has not been produced commercially for many years. Consequently in this entry, as in the routine laboratory, 'Methyl Green' implies the current commercially available Methyl Green (i.e. CI 45290). This molecule contains six methyl and one ethyl substituents. Methyl Green is a hydrophilic, cationic dye, of moderate size.

In this entry, as in the routine laboratory, 'Pyronin' implies Pyronin Y. This is a small, weakly hydrophilic, cationic dye.

Many variants of this method exist. The following procedure may be regarded as typical (but see below). Specimens are stained in an aqueous, slightly acidic, dye-bath containing both Methyl Green and Pyronin. They are then rinsed briefly in water, blotted dry, dehydrated carefully through some organic solvent, and mounted.

This procedure involves basic dyeing. The cationic dyes bind to tissue polyanions. Methyl Green binds preferentially to DNA in chromatin. Pyronin binds preferentially to RNA in ribosomes, and also to anionic glycosaminoglycans, often metachromatically. The nature of the chromatin/ribosome (or DNA/RNA) selectivity remains disputed, but certainly involves competition, as either dye applied singly colors both chromatin and ribosome-rich cytoplasms. One proposed mechanism involves rate control. It is suggested that the smaller, faster diffusing Pyronin stains the less permeable ribosomal sites, whereas the larger, slower diffusing Methyl Green stains the more permeable chromatin. More recent work, however, argues that the preference of Methyl Green for DNA is due to intercalation, with Pyronin binding to single and double-stranded nucleic acids in an indiscriminate manner.

With pure dye samples and a standardized procedure, the relative and absolute dye concentrations in the working solution remain influential, as does the pH and the amount of electrolyte in the dye-bath. With many commercial dye batches of Pyronin, however, the method becomes sensitive to fixation, and more sensitive to other environmental effects. The really significant factor in this case is, therefore, the purity of the Pyronin.

See Plate 17.

Common variants

For almost every aspect of the procedure, some alternative has been recommended: dye concentrations, both absolute and relative; staining temperature and staining time; and the amount and character of co-solutes in the dye-bath. Recommended poststaining procedures are also multitudinous: rinses differ in extent and temperature; and dehydrating regimes are varied. Fortunately, it has been demonstrated that when dyes of reasonable purity are used, and these are now commercially available, standardized staining methods are widely applicable (see Hoyer et al 1986).

AVOIDING PROBLEMS

➤ **What types of specimen processing are suitable?**

The method can be applied to cryosections, paraffin sections and hydrophilic resin sections, sometimes after minor modifications.

▶ Is this procedure easy to carry out?

The method is technically simple, and if pure dyes and a standardized method are used it is straightforward and reliable. If you use low-dye-content Pyronin samples, or 'Pyronin' which is actually rhodamine B, you're on your own.

▶ Obtaining and keeping reliable reagents

1. Commercial samples of Methyl Green are often of high dye content and purity.

2. Contemporary Methyl Green (i.e. CI 42590), unlike the traditional product (i.e. CI 42585), is stable on storage. Consequently, it is advisable to use modern samples.

3. Traditional Methyl Green batches, still on the shelves of many laboratories, may contain excessive amounts of the Crystal Violet contaminant. This may be removed by solvent extraction (e.g. Chayen & Bitensky 1991: 92).

4. For many years commercial Pyronin samples were notoriously impure, with bad effects on the reliability of the Methyl Green–Pyronin method. However, pure material is now commercially available. The colors of pure Pyronin and the dyes sometimes sold in its place are, unfortunately, rather similar. The best advice is to purchase material of high stated dye content. Once a satisfactory material has been obtained, retain a sample for use as a positive reagent control for the next batch of Pyronin purchased.

5. While the Methyl Green–Pyronin stock solution will differ from one variant to another, a weakly acidic stock solution containing both dyes is often stable for several weeks.

▶ Useful control procedures

1. To check that pyroninophilia is due to RNA, insert a prior extraction with 1 M HCl at 60°C for 5 min before staining.

This should remove RNA, but note that remaining DNA may stain red after this treatment. Alternatively, extract the RNA with ribonuclease.

PROBLEMS AND HOW TO DEAL WITH THEM

► **Staining is of an unexpected color**

(*Note*: Such artifacts are exacerbated by impure batches of Pyronin.)

The tissue section may appear too green, for various reasons:

1. Some fixatives can have this effect, try varying the Methyl Green/Pyronin ratio and in future work try using a different fixative.

2. The Pyronin sample used may have been of low dye content. Try increasing the Pyronin content in the working solution.

3. If the poststaining rinse is too short, ribosome-rich cytoplasms may stain greenish-purple. Try extending the rinsing time slightly.

4. Excessive losses of Pyronin can occur into dehydrating fluids, especially if these are ethanolic. Use an agent such as absolute butanol for dehydration.

5. If, when using tissue embedded in hydrophilic resin, there is purple background staining of the resin, check if the Methyl Green is old and contaminated with Crystal Violet (see Horobin et al 1992). If so, use a new batch, or purify by solvent extraction.

The section may appear too pink, for various reasons:

6. Some fixatives can have this effect, try varying the Methyl Green/Pyronin ratio and in future work try using a different fixative.

7. Because an acid decalcification procedure has been used. Try using EDTA, or increasing the proportion of Methyl

Green. (*Note*: Other reports suggest that acid decalcification may make the section stain too greenish a tint!)

8. Excessive losses of Methyl Green can occur into the poststaining rinse. Try reducing the rinsing times or the temperature of the rinse.

9. Excessive losses of Methyl Green can also occur into dehydrating fluids if these are too polar. To limit losses, blot sections dry after the poststaining aqueous rinse.

➤ Other problems

Red cytoplasmic staining is not always due to RNA, and so not all cells with red cytoplasms are plasma cells. Other reasons include:

1. The presence of glycosaminoglycans. If this is a possibility, use acid extraction of RNA as a control procedure (see below). Alternatively, stain in the presence of 0.1 M NaCl, which inhibits staining of glycosaminoglycans by Pyronin but does not inhibit RNA coloration.

2. As the pH rises above 5, the staining of proteins will also rise. Check the pH of the staining solutions.

3. If the pH is below 5, but there is extensive red cytoplasmic staining, the 'Pyronin' used may actually have been Rhodamine B. This can be checked by taking a look at the cytoplasm of cells such as smooth muscle cells. If these are red, discard the dye and obtain a batch of real Pyronin.

Background reading

The statement regarding the commercial availability of Methyl Green is from Green (1990: 458). The rate control theory of Methyl Green–Pyronin staining was set out by Goldstein (1961). More recent affinity-controlled theorizing is summarized by Lyon (1991: 93), whose group earlier dramatically demonstrated the bad effects of Pyronin impurities (Lyon et al 1982).

30 Miller's elastin stain: a modified Weigert technique

Background information

The key staining solution is prepared by heating a solution of three basic dyes (Crystal Violet, New Fuchsin and Victoria Blue R) with ferric chloride and resorcinol. The literature indicates that, under these conditions, cationic dyes with large conjugated systems will be generated from both Crystal Violet and New Fuchsin. Victoria Blue is already a cationic dye with a large conjugated system; whether it is altered by the treatment is not known.

The staining technique involves an initial oxidation of sections with permanganate, followed by removal of manganese dioxide with oxalic acid. The staining solution, in the form of a strongly acid aqueous alcoholic solution, is then applied. Various counterstains may then be applied; in particular picrotrichromes, such as the Van Gieson's and picro-Sirius Red variants (see below).

Affinity for elastin is provided by the large conjugated systems of the dyes present in the staining solution. This feature results in van der Waals forces being enhanced.

Also contributing to binding of these cationic dyes are the sulfonate anions generated from sulfur-containing amino acid residues in elastin by the permanganate oxidation. Staining selectivity is achieved by the use of strongly acidic alcohol as staining solvent. The acidity suppresses ionization of phosphate and carboxylate groups, and so DNA,

RNA and some glycosaminoglycans fail to stain by basic dyeing. The acidity also results in tissue proteins, other than the weakly ionic elastin, being strongly cationic; hence these are not stained by the cationic dyes, despite the enhancement of van der Waals attractions. The alcohol prevents hydrophobic bonding aiding staining of the background.

See Plate 18.

Common variants

The stain may be used undiluted for a few hours, or in diluted form overnight. Ethyl Violet can replace Crystal Violet. Various counterstains (e.g. Van Gieson's or picro-Sirius Red trichromes) may be applied after the staining of elastic fibers.

AVOIDING PROBLEMS

➤ **What types of specimen processing are suitable?**

There appears to be no restriction on which fixative can be used.

➤ **Is this procedure easy to carry out?**

This method is simple and reliable. As it does not require differentiation, it is well suited for identifying fine elastic fibers, which can lose dye if treated with acid alcohol. The staining time is rather long; moreover, the staining solution is time consuming to prepare, although once made has a long shelf-life.

➤ **Obtaining and keeping reliable reagents**

1. The stain does not seem very sensitive to variations in dye content.

2. Use fresh ferric chloride solution, prepared from analytical-grade reagent, when preparing the stain.

3. Once prepared, an effective batch of stain may be used

repeatedly, and if stored in the refrigerator can be used for several weeks.

PROBLEMS AND HOW TO DEAL WITH THEM

➤ Tissue stains unexpectedly weakly

1. This is a rather slow stain, so try extending the staining time. (*Guideline*: if using the undiluted stain, staining for several hours may be required.)

2. When long staining times fail to give strong staining, it is likely that the stain was not prepared successfully. Make up a fresh batch, using fresh ferric chloride solution.

➤ Unexpected structures stain

1. In addition to elastin, a few high-affinity sites (e.g. the sulfated heparin of mast cell granules) are colored with this stain.

Background reading

The original method was described by Miller (1971). Evidence for the chemical structure of the reaction product of New Fuchsin, ferric chloride and resorcinol is available (Horobin et al 1974, Horobin & Flemming 1980, Proctor & Horobin 1988). Discussion of the selective staining of the elastic fibers by cationic dyes with large conjugated systems, applied from acid alcoholic solutions, is available (Horobin & James 1970, Horobin & Flemming 1980).

It has been shown that Victoria Blue R may be used, without ferric reaction with chloride or resorcinol, to selectively stain elastic fibers from acid alcohol (Tsutsumi et al 1990).

31 MSB technique for fibrin and other acidophilic materials

Background information

The standard procedure uses three acid dyes: Martius Yellow, the small anion of which is weakly hydrophilic; Brilliant Crystal Scarlet (synonym: Crystal Ponceau 6R), the anion of which is of moderate size and hydrophilicity; and Methyl Blue (synonyms: Aniline Blue, Soluble Blue), which possesses hydrophilic anions of large size. The method also uses phosphotungstic acid, which possesses hydrophilic anions of large size.

There are both sequence stain and one-bath variants of this staining method. The initial coloration step of the sequence stain uses an alcoholic solution containing Martius Yellow and phosphotungstic acid. Next, an aqueous acidic solution of Brilliant Crystal Scarlet is used, followed by a differentiation step in which the red dye is selectively removed from collagen fibers using phosphotungstic acid. Finally, the collagen is stained with Methyl Blue. Since the solutions used are strongly acidic, prior staining of nuclei with the acid-stable Celestine Blue–hematoxylin is routine.

Each of the anionic dyes used in this method have a non-specific affinity for proteins, since these biopolymers will carry many cationic substituents under the acid conditions used. Staining selectivity is due to competition based on rate control. Thus the different dyes will diffuse at markedly differing rates, the largest being the slowest diffusing, and tissues vary from very permeable (collagen fibers) to poorly permeable (e.g. red blood cells). The outcome is that the erythrocytes stain yellow, and collagen stains blue, with materials of intermediate permeability, such as fibrin, staining red.

See Plate 19.

Common variants

The Martius Yellow can be replaced by Lissamine Fast Yellow. Various red acid dyes of moderate size can substitute for Brilliant Crystal Scarlet, commercially available compounds including Ponceau 2R and Azophloxine. Many large blue or green acid dyes are suitable replacements for Methyl Blue (e.g. Evans Blue, Fast Green FCF or Naphthalene Black 10B, which are commercially available).

As already noted, this method has both one-bath and sequence staining variants.

AVOIDING PROBLEMS

➤ **What types of specimen processing are suitable?**

Best results are obtained with dichromate or other heavy metal fixatives. Routine paraffin sections are used.

➤ **Is this procedure easy to carry out?**

The one-bath variant is easy and reliable. However, although the sequence version can give elegant results, it is difficult for the new or occasional user (see Lillie & Fulmer 1976: 699). In particular note that there are two steps requiring microscopic control.

The methods are routinely carried on paraffin sections, with no particular fixative being recommended. Due to the use of highly acidic solutions, and of dyes in the size range 500–1000 daltons, these methods are not suitable for specimens embedded in glycolmethacrylate resins.

➤ Obtaining and keeping reliable reagents

1. Methyl Blue and Aniline Blue are routinely mixtures of dyes, differing in their degree of phenylation, methylation and sulphonation. There is marked batch variation. However, none of this seems to matter in this procedure.

2. After the working solution has been prepared, it needs to stand for a few days before use, otherwise polychromasia is underdeveloped. After this period it is stable for several weeks.

PROBLEMS AND HOW TO DEAL WITH THEM

➤ Tissue stains unexpectedly weakly

1. If, when using the standard sequence stain, erythrocytes stain red, rather than yellow, try replacing the Martius Yellow with Lissamine Fast Yellow, since this latter, larger dye is more resistant to removal by the subsequent red dye.

➤ Staining is of an unexpected color

1. When using the standard sequence stain, if fibrin that is not suspected to be old stains blue, examine after 2 min, and at 2-min intervals. Alternatively, try replacing the Methyl Blue with Evans Blue, as this larger, slower staining dye will be less likely to replace the red dye in the fibrin.

2. When using the standard sequence stain, if the collagen looks red or purple, rather than blue, extend the phosphotungstic acid differentiation step until all red dye is removed. (*Guideline*: If using a 5-min differentiation, extend to 10 min as a trial.)

3. If polychromasia is weak, check that the working solution has stood for a few days on the bench, and is not freshly prepared.

Background reading

For a general account of this type of rate controlled staining system, see Baker (1958). There you will also find a delightful definition of phosphotungstic acid as 'a colorless acid dye'. Both the sequence and one-bath MSB methods were first described by Lendrum et al (1962). The size criteria underlying successful staining of hydrophilic resins such as glycolmethacrylate, have been discussed (Gerrits et al 1990).

32 Myoadenylate deaminase for muscle-fiber typing

Background information

Key reactants are the substrate adenosine 5'-monophosphate, the visualizing agent Nitro Blue Tetrazolium, and the reducing agent dithiothreitol. In the presence of the substrate the deaminase activity results in the release of ammonia. The resulting high pH permits reduction of the tetrazolium salt to a formazan by the dithiothreitol. The formazan is insoluble and, due to its large conjugated system, binds strongly to tissue proteins.

AVOIDING PROBLEMS

➤ **What types of specimen processing are suitable?**

This method requires fresh cryostat sections, and stained preparations are mounted in glycerin jelly.

➤ **Is this procedure easy to carry out?**

Perhaps the only tricky aspect is the fact that dithiothreitol attacks electrodes, which makes adjusting the pH of the incubation media awkward.

➤ **Obtaining and keeping reliable reagents**

Make up fresh incubating solution each time the method is to be applied. The reagents keep well in the refrigerator.

➤ **Useful routine control procedures**

1. To check that staining is enzymic, substitute inosine 5'-monophosphate for the AMP.

2. Use a positive muscle biopsy control.

PROBLEMS AND HOW TO DEAL WITH THEM

➤ **Tissue stains unexpectedly weakly**

1. This method usually gives weak staining, so do not use thin sections if you wish to see a reaction product.

➤ **Staining is of an unexpected color**

1. If this occurs, prepare a fresh solution of potassium chloride.

➤ **Nature of staining is unusual**

1. If this occurs it is probably due to Nothing dehydrogenase.

Background reading

The use of this procedure to diagnose pathological myoadenylate deaminase deficiency was first discussed by Fishbein et al (1978). An account of its diagnostic application has been given by Dubowitz (1985).

33 NADH diaphorase for muscle biopsies

Background information

The key reactants are reduced nicotine adenine dinucleotide (NADH) plus a tetrazolium salt as an electron acceptor/visualizing agent. The latter may be Nitro Blue Tetrazolium (NBT), a bistetrazolium salt with a large conjugated system, which gives rise to a formazan reaction product that binds well to tissue proteins by van der Waals forces. Alternatively, methylthiazolyldiphenyl tetrazolium (MTT) may be used. The monoformazan which derives from MTT has a smaller conjugated system, with a lower substantivity. However, this may be transformed into a MTT formazan–cobalt chelate by treatment with cobalt ions. This chelate has a larger conjugated system, of higher substantivity.

NADH diaphorase is the enzyme that catalyzes the dehydrogenation of the reduced form of the coenzyme NAD. When this occurs in the presence of a suitable tetrazolium salt, the latter is converted to an insoluble colored formazan.

Common variants

Two commonly used tetrazolium salts are MTT and NBT. The former requires mounting in an aqueous medium, whilst the latter permits dehydration, clearing and mounting in resinous media.

AVOIDING PROBLEMS

➤ What types of specimen processing are suitable?

Unfixed cryostat sections are usually used, with postfixation applied after staining. However, NADH tetrazolium reductase can still be demonstrated after fixation in acetone or formalin.

➤ Is this procedure easy to carry out?

There are no particular problems with this procedure, other than the relatively high cost of MTT. If mounting in glycerin jelly or other water-soluble mounting media, allow the section to dry before mounting, in order to avoid bubble formation.

➤ Obtaining and keeping reliable reagents

1. Commercial samples of NBT may be contaminated by significant amounts of the corresponding monotetrazolium salt, which gives rise to red staining rather than the expected blue coloration. If you wish to check monotetrazolium levels, use a thin layer chromatographic method (see Seidler 1991: 15), or just obtain another batch of reagent from a different supplier, since there is no easy way to remove such impurities.

2. Since MTT is relatively expensive, it is usual to freeze-down aliquots of MTT incubation medium, in which form the salt is stable for several weeks.

PROBLEMS AND HOW TO DEAL WITH THEM

➤ Tissue stains unexpectedly weakly

1. The enzyme can be lost from fresh frozen sections. Add a colloid-protecting agent, such as polyvinylpyrrolidone, to the incubation medium. Alternatively, try fixing in acetone or formalin prior to staining.

➤ Unexpected structures stain

1. Direct reduction of tetrazolium salts is possible under

alkaline conditions. Check that incubation was indeed carried out at neutral pH.

2. NBT can give rise to crystalline precipitates on the surface of fat droplets. Ignore these.

➤ Staining is of an unexpected color

1. NBT can give rise to pink-purple staining, especially if the enzyme levels are low. This is either due to reduction to the half formazan, or to the presence of excessive contamination by the monotetrazolium salt (see above); the matter is disputed. In either event, this effect can be ignored, or you may remove the formazan from the sections by washing with acetone.

Background reading

Some of the biochemical aspects of these histochemical methods are discussed by Chayen & Bitensky (1991, see especially pp. 225–237).

34 Nonspecific esterase using an azodye method

Background information

The method requires two key reagents: the synthetic organic carboxyester, α-naphthyl acetate, as a substrate; and a diazonium salt as visualizing agent. Both Fast Blue B or Hexazotized Pararosanilin have been recommended; the latter having a relatively large conjugated system.

Esterases catalyze the hydrolysis of the substrate, yielding α-naphthol. In this simultaneous coupling procedure, the colorless α-naphthol reaction product is visualized by its conversion into an insoluble azodye, by reaction with the diazonium salt. Esterases hydrolyze short-chain fatty acid esters preferentially, while long-chain fatty acid esters are preferentially hydrolyzed by lipases. Cholinesterases attack choline esters selectively. All these enyzmes give rise to staining with this method, hence the description 'nonspecific' esterase.

Precise cellular localization of stain, and resistance to extraction into solvents and mountants, is favored by using a visualizing agent with a larger conjugated system (i.e. Hexazotized Pararosanilin), as this enhances azodye–protein binding.

See Plate 20.

Common variants

Diazonium salt visualizing agents may be a stabilized fast salt (routinely Fast Blue B) or freshly prepared Hexazotized Pararosanilin. When the latter is used sections can be mounted in resin, otherwise an aqueous mountant is required.

AVOIDING PROBLEMS

➤ What types of specimen processing are suitable?

Frozen sections are usually recommended, prefixed in formalin or formaldehyde vapor. However, activity is retained even in formalin-fixed paraffin sections at some sites. Staining specimens embedded in glycolmethacrylate resin gives excellent results.

➤ Is this procedure easy to carry out?

If carried out using Fast Blue as visualizing agent, this method is straightforward. The method can be carried out on cryosections, and when Hexazotized Pararosanilin is used (see below) may be applied to glycolmethacrylate resin sections without modification.

Preparation of the working solution of Fast Blue is simple, but this visualizing agent necessitates the use of an aqueous mountant. Preparation of Hexazotized Pararosanilin is more troublesome, but permits mounting in, superior, resin systems.

The reaction time can be rapid, so do not overstain.

➤ Obtaining and keeping reliable reagents

1. Commercial diazonium (i.e. 'fast') salts contain stabilizer, and can be stored long-term in the refrigerator.

2. However, make up the solutions freshly for each stain, since once dissolved the salts quickly deteriorate.

3. For the same reason, prepare solutions of Hexazotized Pararosanilin freshly for each investigation.

4. In addition, ensure that sodium nitrite solutions used for diazotization of the Pararosanilin are freshly prepared from recently opened containers.

➤ Useful routine control procedures

1. Staining should be totally prevented by enzyme inactivation (heat in boiling water for 10 min), or by omitting the substrate from the incubation solution.

PROBLEMS AND HOW TO DEAL WITH THEM

➤ Tissue stains unexpectedly weakly

1. Diazonium salts are unstable in solution. Make sure they are dissolved or prepared immediately prior to incubating the slide.

➤ Unexpected structures stain

1. Selectivity requires use of a low pH. Check the pH of the incubation medium and, if necessary, adjust it downwards.

2. Sulfated glycosaminoglycans (e.g. those in mucus goblet cells) may give false-positive staining due to binding of diazonium salts. This is nonenzymic, and so will be detected by routine control procedure 1 (see above).

➤ Staining is of an unexpected color

1. A generalized background staining of a different color to that expected, and perhaps seen, at enzymic sites can arise from reaction of the diazonium salt with tissue proteins. Ignore such background staining.

Background reading

A good account of the histochemical implications of the rather complex biochemistry of esterases is provided by Chayen & Bitensky (1991).

35 Nile Blue sulfate for neutral and acidic lipids

Background information

Aqueous solutions of Nile Blue contain a slightly lipophilic blue cation plus its free base. A red nonionic, lipophilic decomposition product, Nile Red, is also routinely present. The amount of this latter dye increases in a heated, acidic solution. For the method to be effective, the presence of Nile Red is essential.

The procedure involves the following steps. Prepare an acidic working solution by boiling Nile Blue with dilute aqueous sulfuric acid. Stain with a hot acidic Nile Blue solution. Differentiate for a couple of minutes with dilute aqueous acetic acid. Mount in an aqueous medium.

The Nile Red dissolves in all lipid components, staining them pink. Nile Blue cations bind to anionic groups in the tissues, the carboxylic groups of fatty acids, and phosphate groups of phospholipids giving a blue coloration. Basic dyeing of nonlipid components is inhibited by the low pH used. The acidic aqueous differentiator removes Nile Blue selectively from the more hydrophilic nonlipid sites.

Sensitivity is dependent on the amount of Nile Red in the Nile Blue, and on the overall concentration of dye used. As Nile Red only penetrates liquid lipids, sensitivity of neutral lipid staining is also dependent on staining temperature. Selectivity is influenced by pH, acidic solutions being needed for selectivity. The poststaining acetic acid wash can also affect staining, since it can nonselectively remove excessive amounts of dye.

Common variants

There are a number of related methods in the literature, and the terminology describing them has become confused.

Some methods use commercial batches of Nile Blue, and assume there is sufficient Nile Red present as a contaminant. Variants ensure the necessary Nile Red content in various ways. The specific method described in this entry achieves this by boiling a dilute sulfuric acid solution of Nile Blue before staining. Variants use dye prepared specifically for this method, such that the contamination of the dye is guaranteed, or add Nile Red to the Nile Blue.

The staining procedures of the variants also differ. Thus recommended dye concentrations vary, as do staining and differentiating temperatures, and staining pH. Use of acidic poststaining differentiation also varies.

AVOIDING PROBLEMS

➤ **What types of specimen processing are suitable?**

It is typically carried out on cryosections, since some lipids will be extracted during paraffin embedding or de-waxing. However, fatty acids that are present as their soaps, following calcium formal fixation, commonly survive in paraffin sections.

➤ **Is this procedure easy to carry out?**

The method is straightforward, and requires no special skill.

➤ **Useful control procedures**

1. As a positive control for the efficacy of Nile Red staining of neutral lipids, stain a test section of material known to contain fatty connective tissue.

2. To check if blue staining is due to the presence of phospholipids, saponify fatty acids by prior acid hydrolysis, wash and dry the sections, and then extract free fatty acids with cold acetone prior to staining with the Nile Blue sulfate procedure. For details, see Bancroft & Stevens (1996: 221).

PROBLEMS AND HOW TO DEAL WITH THEM

➤ Stain or staining solution not as expected

1. Nile Blue is commonly supplied as the sulfate, although the less soluble chloride has also been sold. The latter may give rise to solubility problems. However, in the variant discussed in this entry, dye should dissolve on being refluxed with dilute sulfuric acid.

➤ Tissue stains unexpectedly weakly

1. Weak staining of neutral lipids occurs if the dye batch does not contain sufficient Nile Red. Check this by using the positive control for Nile Red (see above).

2. If Nile Red is present in a reasonable amount, but staining of neutral lipids is nevertheless weak or absent, check the temperature of the dye-bath, and try raising it to 70°C.

3. Weak staining of fatty acids or phospholipids can result from overdifferentiation following staining. If this is suspected, try shortening the acetic acid wash.

4. Nile Blue readily fades, so keep stained slides out of sunlight and preferably observe them soon after staining.

➤ Unexpected structures stain

1. Blue background or nuclear staining may occur if the pH of the working solution rises. Check the pH, it should be at 2.

Background reading

Much has been published concerning the variants of this method. A straightforward and critical account is given by Dunnigan (1968a,b).

36 Oil Red O for fats

Background information

Oil Red O is a nonionic, hydrophobic dye of moderate size. This dye gives intense staining of the triglycerides of fats, but is a markedly less effective stain for phospholipids. A generalized technical protocol follows.

Staining is carried out using saturated or supersaturated solutions of the dye in aqueous–organic solvent mixtures. Background staining is removed by differentiation with dye-free solvent. An optional prestaining bromination step can be used to enhance staining of free fatty acids and lecithin, but not of cholesterol.

Staining involves a partitioning process. Hydrophobic dye moves from the relatively polar solvent into nonaqueous, lipid-containing regions of the specimen. The hydrated parts of the sections have only a low affinity for the dye, and any which does enter is removed by the differentiator. High-melting lipids, such as crystalline cholesterol deposits, will not stain.

Sensitivity is strongly influenced by the solvent. Lipid can be extracted from the specimen during staining, and the solvent's polarity controls dye partitioning. Moreover, since saturated solutions of Oil Red O are used, the concentration depends on the solvent's ability to dissolve dye. Sensitivity is also influenced by access of stain to the lipid, with solid and especially crystalline lipids failing to stain. Sensitivity is substantially influenced by the differentiation step and the polarity of the solvent.

See Plate 21.

Common variants

The routine dye solvent is 70% alcohol. To increase dye concentrations, and hence staining intensity, alternative solvents such as isopropanol, triethylphosphate and propylene glycol may be used. Suggested staining times range widely, from 2 h with the lower dye concentrations to 10 min in the better solvents. To increase staining sensitivity, bromination pretreatment may be used.

AVOIDING PROBLEMS

➤ **What types of specimen processing are suitable?**

The method uses unfixed or briefly fixed cryosections, since lipids are lost during paraffin embedding and de-waxing.

➤ **Is this procedure easy to carry out?**

This is a straightforward method.

➤ **Obtaining and keeping reliable reagents**

1. Commercial samples of Oil Red O routinely contain small amounts of several isomers and homologs.

2. Stock solutions of saturated Oil Red O in isopropanol or triethylphosphate are stable indefinitely.

➤ **Useful control procedures**

1. As a routine control, stain a section that has been de-lipidized by extraction with chloroform–methanol. This solvent removes all lipids, and so any Oil Red O staining will be artifactual.

PROBLEMS AND HOW TO DEAL WITH THEM

➤ Tissue stains unexpectedly weakly

1. Methods that use 70% alcohol as solvent, with staining times longer than 30 min, may extract lipid from the section into the dye-bath. Try shorter staining times. If this does not help, try using a supersaturated solution of Oil Red O in isopropanol or triethylphosphate, for a shorter time.

➤ Unexpected structures stain

1. If the background is difficult to decolorize, check the temperature of the poststaining wash. If it is too cold, too little dye is removed.

➤ Nature of staining is unusual

1. Aggregation of fat droplets into larger drops is encouraged both by the use of triethylphosphate as the solvent and by bromination. If such aggregation occurs, and is confusing, avoid such procedures.

2. Although the better dye solvents can result in more intense staining, such high dye concentrations do increase the chances of dye crystallizing in fat deposits on storage. If this occurs, reduce the intensity of staining.

➤ Other problems

1. Oil Red O can precipitate from the supersaturated solutions onto the sections. To minimize this, filter solutions just before use, and always use a covered container when staining in order to minimize alcohol evaporation. It has been suggested that adding 1% dextrin to the aqueous solvent component stabilizes the Oil Red O solution.

Background reading

For background discussion of the method and its variants, and technical details of the procedures noted in this entry, see Bayliss High (1990).

37 Papanicolaou stains for cytology

Background information

Papanicolaou stains all use two acid dyes (Light Green SF and Eosin Y), and some variants use three (Orange G). The size of these hydrophilic, anionic dyes decreases from Light Green to Orange G. Working solutions containing these dyes also contain phosphotungstate anions. Most Papanicolaou variants use hematoxylin as the nuclear counterstain, although one standardized method uses Thionin (a small, hydrophilic cationic dye). Traditional Papanicolaou formulations often contained Bismark Brown; this is not discussed here because it does not in fact stain the specimens.

The first step stains nuclei and basophilic cytoplasms. If Orange G is used, this is applied next, in an alcoholic solution containing phosphotungstate. The mixture of Eosin and Light Green is then applied, again in alcoholic solution with phosphotungstate present. At this stage Orange G is largely replaced by Eosin in more keratinized cells, and by Light Green in less keratinized sites, leaving the smaller dye in hyperkeratinized cells, nucleoli, and so on.

Papanicolaou staining involves acid and basic dyeing. Basic dye cations stain DNA and RNA polyanions; acid dye anions stain proteins, these being polycationic in the acidic dye-baths used. Since keratin is less permeable than other cellular proteins, and since the larger a dye the slower it diffuses, the acid dye polychromasia is influenced by rate effects. The progressively more keratinized cells are stained preferentially by the increasingly smaller dyes. The sites of uptake and the relative amounts of Eosin and Light Green bound are also dependent on the solution's acidity and on the amount of phosphotungstate present. This latter reagent also retains the basic dye, in the subsequent alcoholic dye-baths, as basic dye-phosphotungstate salts are insoluble in both alcohol and water.

Staining intensities of the acid dyes are influenced by dye-bath acidity, and those of basic dyes are influenced by counterstaining by trapping with phosphotungstate (but see also Entry 22, 'Hematoxylin and Eosin as an oversight stain'). Selective acid dye coloration also depends on the acidity, as well as the specimen shape (e.g. thinness of smear and cell type).

See Plate 22.

Common variants

There are many variants. Some omit dyes (often Bismark Brown, sometimes Orange G), some use alternative dyes (e.g. hematoxylin has been replaced by Thionin, and Light Green by Fast Green), and phosphomolybdate is sometimes substituted for phosphotungstate. The solvent used in the Eosin–Light Green dye-bath varies; 50% and 70% aqueous ethanol solutions are both recommended. The preferred acidity of this solution also varies in the range pH 4–6. (*Note*: These solutions are substantially nonaqueous, so it is more accurate to say 'apparent pH'.)

AVOIDING PROBLEMS

➤ What types of specimen processing are suitable?

Specimens are typically smears, wet-fixed with ethanol. However, with suitable modifications, paraffin or celloidin sections can also be used, as can many fixation regimes, with ethanol–ether, propanol and formaldehyde systems all having their protagonists.

▶ Is this procedure easy to carry out?

The method is complicated and specimen dependent. However, routine, even standardized, versions can be developed.

▶ Obtaining and keeping reliable reagents

1. All the dyes used in the Papanicolaou method are available commercially in reasonably pure form.

2. The solutions of the acid dyes (i.e. Orange G and the mixture of Eosin and Light Green) in phosphotungstate-containing ethanol are stable indefinitely.

PROBLEMS AND HOW TO DEAL WITH THEM

▶ Tissue stains unexpectedly weakly

1. Is overall staining weak? If so, check whether specimens were spray-fixed using a polyethylene glycol (PEG)–ethanol mixture. The protective polymer may not have been completely removed prior to staining. Extend prestaining washing with aqueous ethanol, or residual PEG may block access of dyes to the specimen.

2. Is nuclear staining weak? If alcohol fixation was used, check the fixation time. If less than 15 min, try extending the time. For other possible causes of weak staining by hematoxylin, see entry 22, 'Hematoxylin and Eosin as an oversight stain'.

3. Does the green coloration fade? If so, replace Light Green with the more stable Fast Green.

▶ Staining is of an unexpected color

1. If you look at preparations stained in a laboratory other than your own, remember that Papanicolaou stains have no 'authorized' color balance, and different laboratories favor different colors.

2. If using variants containing Orange G, then orange over-

staining of the centres of cell clumps may be due to slow penetration of the larger eosin and Light Green dyes. Attempt to prepare smears as monolayers.

3. Even in variants not containing Orange G, orange staining occurs, due to Eosin. In such procedures, if entities such as parakeratotic cells infected with human papilloma virus, or malignant squamous cells, fail to stain orange, check the composition of the solvent, and adjust if necessary. Use of 95% ethanol suppresses such orange Eosin staining, while 50% ethanol permits it.

4. Staining that is too green can arise for various reasons:

   (a) If red-stained nucleoli are required, check the apparent pH. If necessary, use a Papanicolaou stain with an apparent pH higher than 6.0.

   (b) If the specimen was stained on a Friday, when was the working solution prepared, and has it been heavily used? Repeated use of a working solution depletes the Eosin faster than the Light Green.

► Other problems

1. Capricious staining can arise if a smear preparation is not in monolayer form. Look to see if numerous cell clumps are present. If so, attempt to prepare future smears as monolayers. Since the staining is substantially rate controlled, these will be less variable in staining than will clumps of irregular size. Are smears prepared manually, or with a device such as a cytocentrifuge? If manually, consider using an automated system.

Background reading

An overview of the principles and practice of Papanicolaou stains is available (Boon & Druijver, 1986). Standardization and quantification of Papanicolaou staining are discussed in a book edited by Boon & Kok (1986). For evidence that Bismark Brown does not contribute to staining, see Marshall et al (1979).

38 The periodic acid–Schiff (PAS) procedure for polysaccharides

Background information

Key reagents in the PAS procedure are the selective oxidant periodic acid, and the Schiff reagent. The latter is a solution containing a colorless derivative of Basic Fuchsin, in which a sulfite moiety has been attached to the central carbon atom. Satisfactory Schiff reagent can be prepared from either of the commercially available homologues of Basic Fuchsin (pararosanilin and New Fuchsin). Other necessary components of Schiff reagent are hydrogen ions and sulfite ions.

The PAS procedure for demonstrating polysaccharides involves an initial generation of aldehyde groups, by oxidation of suitable glycol fragments in the biopolymers by the periodic acid. The aldehydes are subsequently converted to Schiff reagent derivatives. These initial reaction products are colorless, but are converted to magenta final reaction products by the post-Schiff-reagent washing steps.

Sensitivity and selectivity are consequently dependent on several factors. Highly water-soluble polysaccharides must be retained in the specimen during processing and staining. Polysaccharides must contain glycol fragments, which rapidly oxidize to aldehydes. Endogenous aldehyde groups should be absent. The Schiff reagent must not decompose during staining.

See Plate 23.

Common variants

The variants of the PAS procedure, whilst possessing the characteristics alluded to above, differ as follows.

With regard to the nature of the oxidant and the oxidation step, periodic acid may be used as such, or be produced via the use of an acidified solution of a periodate salt. However, neither the pH nor the effective molar periodic acid concentrations vary significantly between different procedures. The solvent is usually aqueous, although some methods use alcohol. The recommended times and temperatures of oxidation also vary somewhat.

With regard to the composition of the Schiff reagent and the nature of staining process, the source and concentration of sulfite and hydrogen ions may vary. However, bisulfite or metabisulfite ions plus a mineral acid are routine. In any event, the solutions are always strongly acidic, and contain excess sulfite over that needed to react with the Basic Fuchsin. The molar concentrations of this dye are similar in the different methods. The temperatures and times of treatment with Schiff reagent vary.

AVOIDING PROBLEMS

➤ **What types of specimen processing are suitable?**

This method is routinely applied to formalin-fixed paraffin sections. However, there is no overriding fixative dependence, and many other fixatives have been used successfully. Note, however, that if seeking to demonstrate glycogen, alcoholic fixatives retain this water-soluble biopolymer particularly well. The procedure can be applied to tissues embedded in hydrophilic resin media.

➤ **Is this procedure easy to carry out?**

The PAS procedure has no significant difficulties for the average benchworker.

➤ Obtaining and keeping reliable reagents

1. At the time of writing, standardized Schiff reagent is not commercially available. However, since a simple procedure for preparing stable, dry Schiff reagent is now available (Galassi 1993), this situation may improve.

2. In the interim, only use colorless samples of Schiff reagent (see below for tips on the recognition of contamination and decomposition).

3. Store Schiff reagent in a tightly sealed bottle, in a refrigerator.

➤ Useful control procedures

1. Stain a specimen omitting the periodate oxidation step. Native or artifactual aldehydes (i.e. nonspecific materials) will be colored purple.

2. Insert an aldehyde blockade after the postoxidation wash and before treatment with Schiff reagent (Bancroft & Stevens 1990: 104). Staining of this control indicates staining due to nonaldehyde materials.

PROBLEMS AND HOW TO DEAL WITH THEM

➤ Stain or staining solution not as expected

1. If the Schiff's reagent looks yellow-brown, this suggests contamination by acridines. Use another batch of reagent; or try de-colorizing with activated charcoal as in the initial preparation of the reagent.

2. If the Schiff reagent is pink tinged and smells only weakly of sulfur dioxide (care!) it may be overaged, as Basic Fuchsin is slowly formed on standing. Use fresh reagent, or reconstitute with bisulfite (see Chung & Chen 1970).

➤ Tissue stains unexpectedly weakly

1. Water-soluble polysaccharides may have been extracted from the specimen into aqueous fixatives. Try fixing spec-

imens in picric–formaldehyde (Chayen & Bitensky 1991: 102) or alcoholic media.

2. Water-soluble polysaccharides may have been extracted into aqueous staining reagents. Try using an alcoholic PAS procedure.

3. Tissue polysaccharides containing anionic polysaccharides and glycosaminoglycans often fail to stain, or stain weakly, after a standard PAS procedure. Try lengthening the oxidation step, or adding magnesium chloride to the periodate solution (Scott & Dorling 1969).

▶ **Unexpected structures stain**

1. Pink background staining may be due to decomposition of Schiff reagent. This can occur for several reasons:

   (a) Aging (see above).

   (b) Carryover of periodate. Try more extended washing following oxidation.

   (c) Thermal decomposition during microwave-accelerated staining. If the stain becomes transiently pink during staining, reduce the time or temperature setting on the oven.

2. Pink background staining also occurs due to artifactual tissue aldehyde groups. These arise in several ways:

   (a) Acrolein or glutaraldehyde fixation. Try another fixative, or treat sections with borohydride prior to oxidation (Bancroft & Stevens 1990: 234).

   (b) Insufficient washing of tissue following formaldehyde fixation. Try extending the wash time.

   (c) In cryosections, aldehydes may be generated from plasmalogen phospholipids by fixatives containing mercuric chloride. Try another fixative.

   (d) The presence of ozone due to photolysis of periodate

(especially sodium periodate) solution. Keep solutions out of direct sunlight.

(e) Lipid-rich material, such as myelin, can be oxidized by periodate, becoming Schiff-positive. Try extracting the section with chloroform–methanol prior to oxidation, and see if staining is now negative.

3. Localized purple or red staining of 'nontarget' structures can occur for various reasons:

(a) Deposits of carbonates and other salts can decompose the Schiff reagent. This can be detected by the routine control 2 (see above).

(b) Cysteine-rich sites, such as hair shafts, may be oxidized by periodate, becoming Schiff-positive (but see comments by Lillie & Fulmer 1976: 230).

4. Intracellular locations of PAS staining can vary with the fixation method used. Try varying the fixative agent or fixative method.

➤ **Staining is of an unexpected color**

1. Yellow-brown background staining may be due to contamination of the Schiff reagent with acridines (see above).

Background reading

The structure and staining mechanism of Schiff reagent is now clear (Robins et al 1980). That satisfactory Schiff reagent can be prepared from pararosanilin or New Fuchsin has been demonstrated by Teichman et al (1980). The size and hydrophilicity criteria underlying successful staining of hydrophilic resins, such as glycolmethacrylate, have been discussed (Gerrits et al 1990, Horobin et al 1991). From a troubleshooting perspective, a useful account of the PAS procedure is that given by Chayen & Bitensky (1991: 99).

39 Perls' Prussian Blue for ferric iron

Background information

The critical reactant is the hexaferrocyanate anion, $Fe(CN)_6^{4-}$. This is applied to sections in the form of an acidic aqueous potassium ferrocyanide (i.e. potassium hexaferrocyanate) solution.

Free ferric ions react with the hexaferrocyanate anions, yielding the brightly colored, insoluble pigment Prussian Blue. Most ferric iron in the tissues is complexed with proteins, in hemoglobin, myoglobin and hemosiderin. Iron is least tightly bound to the latter; at the acidic pH used for staining it is released, and so is free to react.

To demonstrate ferric iron in the other sites, more rigorous pretreatments are called for (e.g. with hydrogen peroxide). To demonstrate ferric oxide, which can occur in tissues due to industrial exposure, higher concentrations of acid are needed. Ferrous iron does not form an insoluble complex under the reaction conditions used, and so is not demonstrated.

Sensitivity is influenced by retention of iron in the tissues, and also by staining conditions, including pH, temperature and staining time. The major influence on sensitivity is perhaps iron contamination of reagents or glassware.

See Plate 24.

Common variants

This procedure has a single crucial step, using a working solution containing only two reagents. Nevertheless, the nature and concentration of the acid used, and the time and temperature of staining, all vary between currently recommended methods.

AVOIDING PROBLEMS

➤ **What types of specimen processing are suitable?**

This method may be used after most types of nonacidic fixative; and with paraffin, cryogenic and hydrophilic resin embedding regimes. Note that extended staining times may be required for the latter.

➤ **Is this procedure easy to carry out?**

This method is straightforward, presenting no difficulties for the routine user.

➤ **Obtaining and keeping reliable reagents**

1. To avoid iron contamination, always use analytical-grade reagents and ensure the use of iron-free water and uncontaminated glassware.

2. Since the acidic ferrocyanide solution is unstable, prepare the working solution freshly before use.

➤ **Useful control procedures**

1. Since iron contamination (of the specimen, reagent or glassware) occurs easily, and as the reagent is unstable, always stain a positive control alongside the experimental specimen.

2. A simple negative control can be obtained by extracting iron from a section (e.g. using oxalic or sulfuric acid) prior to staining.

Individual staining procedures

PROBLEMS AND HOW TO DEAL WITH THEM

► **Tissue stains unexpectedly weakly**

1. Whenever you are surprised by weak staining, or a failure to stain, look at your positive control (see above) as a check that there is nothing wrong with the reagents or the procedure.

2. Low iron concentrations give pale staining. Try extending the staining time. If, however, you extend staining times above 30 min, replace the working solution after that time.

3. Acidic fixation in acidic media may cause loss of iron. Try other media in future work.

4. Failure to demonstrate the ferric iron of myoglobin or hemoglobin, or in ferric oxide, can be due to the loss of the highly water-soluble hydrated ferric iron from the specimen during the pretreatments necessary to release the cation from its complexed state. Explore shorter pretreatment times.

5. It has been suggested that, since ferrocyanide ions diffuse slower than hydrogen ions, acid-induced losses of iron can be reduced by pretreating the section with potassium ferrocyanide solution prior to staining with the acidified ferrocyanide reagent.

6. If the section was stained more than a year or two ago, the staining may have faded. If permanent preparations are called for, carry out a diaminobenzidine (DAB) stain (as in DAB peroxidase procedures) after the ferrocyanide staining and before any counterstain. This produces a brown, nonfading DAB polymer around the Prussian Blue deposits.

► **Unexpected structures stain**

1. Iron contamination is one possible source of false-positives. This can arise from the reagents (see control procedure 1, above), glassware or water. Check glass-

washing procedures and the water source. When applying a group of stains to a liver biopsy always do the Perls' stain first, in order to avoid contamination with iron alum used in the reticulin methods.

2. A finely granular blue deposit, throughout the section, can arise with variants involving staining at elevated temperatures. Use a low temperature method, if necessary with an extended staining time.

3. Do not use a strongly staining control section, as some leaching of the blue reaction product may occur and contaminate the test section, and false-positives may be seen.

➤ **Other problems**

1. If iron is abundant, the procedures suggested in staining manuals may result in overstaining, obscuring surrounding tissue elements. Should this occur, reduce staining times.

Background reading

This method is one of the earliest histochemical procedures, Perls published his version in 1967. For an illuminating account of the difficulties involved in its critical use, see the entry for iron in the monograph by Lillie & Fulmer (1976).

40 Phloxine–Tartrazine technique for viral inclusions

Background information

This method uses two anionic dyes. One is Phloxine, a red, acid dye possessing a lipophilic anion with a substantial conjugated system. The other dye is Tartrazine, a yellow, acid dye with a smaller, and strongly hydrophilic, anion.

Initially all tissues are stained red using Phloxine. Overstained sections are then differentiated under microscopic control, using a solution of Tartrazine in Cellosolve (i.e. 2-ethoxyethanol). The red color is removed first from connective tissue, and then from muscle, leaving viral inclusions red.

In the initial step, Phloxine binds nonselectively, probably both due to acid dyeing to tissue proteins and to van der Waals attractions favored by the large conjugated system of the Phloxine. The second staining step involves the selective replacement of Phloxine by Tartrazine. It seems that this is largely controlled by rate effects. Thus Phloxine is lost fastest from collagen, the most permeable of acidophilic structures, and most slowly from chemically diverse dense structures (e.g. elastin fibers, the cornified layer, Paneth cell granules and Russell bodies).

In keeping with this rate model, Phloxine may be substituted by the larger fluorescein dye Rose Bengal. The smaller fluorescein dyes Erythrosin and Eosin Y are too easily removed by the Tartrazine to be practical substitutes.

See Plate 25.

Common variants

It has been suggested that better contrast is obtained if an alternative pair of dyes are used, namely Rose Bengal and Bismark Brown (Clark 1979).

AVOIDING PROBLEMS

➤ **What types of specimen processing are suitable?**

The procedure can be carried out on paraffin sections, and the fixative type is not critical.

➤ **Is this procedure easy to carry out?**

Except for the differentiation step, which must be carried out under microscopic control, this method presents no practical problems. When interpreting the outcomes, however, remember that a number of structures additional to viral inclusions retain Phloxine.

➤ **Obtaining and keeping reliable reagents**

1. Phloxine and Rose Bengal are routinely mixtures of homologs. However, this has little significance when carrying out this procedure.

2. The Phloxine solution is stable in a Coplin jar at room temperature for many months, despite its high salt content.

➤ **Useful control procedures**

1. As a positive control for the efficacy of Phloxine–Tartrazine staining of viral inclusions, stain a test section of material known to contain such material.

PROBLEMS AND HOW TO DEAL WITH THEM

➤ **Tissue stains unexpectedly weakly**

1. If the background staining by Tartrazine is absent or very pale, check if the post-Tartrazine alcoholic rinse contained more than 5% water. The yellow dye is extremely water soluble, and is readily extracted.

2. If the inclusion bodies of the positive control (see above) stain palely, or fail to stain, repeat the staining procedure taking care, over the differentiation step. It is possible to overdifferentiate and remove all the Phloxine from the inclusion.

➤ **Unexpected structures stain**

1. This method is not specific for viral inclusions. When interpreting the staining results, remember that a variety of intracellular inclusions (e.g. secretion granules and Russell bodies) will also stain red.

Background reading

The consequences of using alternative fluorescein dyes in the Phloxine–Tartrazine stain were noted in the original publication concerning this method (Lendrum 1947). The rate control of sequence acid dyeing has been considered by Baker (1958). The role of van der Waals forces in enhancing the nonionic binding of Phloxine was mentioned by Horobin & Bennion (1973). For indications that the actual mechanism of staining may be more complex than suggested above, see Clark (1979).

41 Phosphorylase for muscle-fiber typing

Background information

These methods require several essential reagents: glucose 1-phosphate, adenosine triphosphate (ATP), glycogen and magnesium chloride in the incubation medium; and an iodine/iodide solution, the active species of which is the tri-iodide anion, as the visualizing agent.

In vivo, the usual role of phosphorylase is to catalyze the hydrolysis of amylose or glycogen to generate glucose. However, the enzyme also catalyzes the reverse reaction, namely the synthesis of amylose and glycogen from glucose. The enzymic steps of this procedure involve the polymerization of the glucose 1-phosphate. The first product is an unbranched polymer, amylose. When inhibitors, such as ethanol, fluoride and mercuric ions, of the branching enzyme are absent from the incubation solution, the enzyme acts on the amylose to form the branched biopolymer, glycogen. These phosphorylative polymerizations are magnesium activated, require ATP as a phosphate source, and need the presence of preformed glycogen as primer.

Visualization of the resulting amylose or glycogen is carried out by the formation of colored complexes between the tri-iodide ion and the polysaccharides. This gives rise to blue and red-brown products respectively.

See Plate 26.

AVOIDING PROBLEMS

➤ What types of specimen processing are suitable?

Unfixed cryostat sections are required. It has been suggested that free-floating sections are preferable, although mounted sections are generally used. Poststaining washes in aqueous alcohol or postfixation in ethanol are sometimes used.

➤ Is this procedure easy to carry out?

The stain fades within a day or less, and if the specimens are to be stored then the final preparation must be wet-mounted in a medium containing tri-iodide.

The stock solutions last for a considerable time. They should be re-frozen after preparing the working solution.

➤ Useful routine control procedures

1. Tissues such as muscle, a routine specimen in the application of this procedure in histopathology, often contains endogenous glycogen. Pretreat sections with diastase to remove this. Alternatively, stain an unincubated section with the iodine/iodide visualization agent.

2. Postincubation treatment with diastase can be used to check that the color is indeed due to glycogen.

3. To distinguish the activities of phosphorylase and branching enzyme, add ethanol and fluoride ion to the incubation medium, as these act as inhibitors of the branching enzyme. After such additions, only blue-stained amylose, arising from the action of phosphorylase, should be seen.

PROBLEMS AND HOW TO DEAL WITH THEM

➤ Tissue stains unexpectedly weakly

1. Tissues not containing native glycogen require addition of the biopolymer to the incubation medium, as a primer. Check that primer was used.

2. Phosphorylase is fixative sensitive. Avoid fixation.

3. Loss of enzyme from the unfixed sections can be inhibited by use of polyvinylpyrrolidone as a colloid-protecting agent. Check that this agent was used. (*Note*: This agent has been said to give rise to an erratic distribution of staining.)

4. Phosphorylase activity can be enhanced by adding insulin to the incubation medium.

5. Adhesion of the glycogen reaction product to the tissue section has been found to be enhanced by leaving the cryosection to stand at room temperature for 10 min before incubating.

6. The glycogen reaction product can be lost into aqueous postincubation rinses. Try using an aqueous ethanolic rinse, or even a postincubation ethanolic fixation.

7. The staining will fade on standing, typically in 12–24 h. How much time elapsed before you viewed the specimen? It has been suggested that fading can be slowed by a poststaining fixation, dehydration and clearing (Sawyer et al 1965).

Background reading

An account of the underlying biochemistry, and its histochemical implications, is provided by Chayen & Bitensky (1991: 201–204). An account of the applications of this procedure has been given by Dubowitz (1985).

42 Phosphotungstic acid hematoxylin (PTAH)

Background information

The staining solution is prepared by reacting hematin with phosphotungstic acid (PTA), yielding a strongly acid solution containing both blue and red anionic species. The hematin may be introduced as such, or generated in situ from hematoxylin. The structures of the staining species are uncertain. However, one interpretation of the observations is that the red complex comprises a large phosphotungstic acid–hematin species, whereas the blue complex is a smaller 2 : 1 hematin–tungstate compound.

The staining procedure involves an initial oxidation of the section with permanganate, or dichromate followed by permanganate when the fixative used does not itself contain dichromate. Note that dichromate typically increases binding of anionic dyes to proteins. Precipitates of manganese dioxide are removed with oxalic acid. Staining in the PTAH solution follows. Although the details of staining differ from one variant to another, the overall picture is that collagen stains red and cell cytoplasms largely stain blue.

Metachromasia due to non-collagen-tissue ligands binding to tungsten of the dye complexes, and polychromasia due to differential rate effects or to hydrogen bonding between the stain and collagen fibrils have all been invoked to explain the staining pattern. However, if the above chemical suggestions are correct, then a rate-control mechanism does appear plausible. Coloration by the large red PTA species would be limited to the most permeable structures, namely the collagen fibers. Less permeable structures would stain with the smaller, faster diffusing, blue dye.

A wide variety of observations are in keeping with this. For instance, a common feature of diverse treatments that increase staining by the red dye (e.g. alkaline hydrolysis, methylation and 6 M urea) is that they increase the permeability of tissues. Again, the rapid and selective loss of the red coloration from stained sections under alkaline conditions is congruent with decomposition of phosphotungstate into simple tungstate ions by strong bases.

See Plate 27.

Common variants

Some variants of the staining solution are prepared directly from hematin; others involve the in situ oxidation of hematoxylin with permanganate or atmospheric oxygen.

AVOIDING PROBLEMS

➤ **What types of specimen processing are suitable?**

Although this method is routinely applied to paraffin sections, it has also been recommended for cryosections. Various fixatives may be used; however, these do give somewhat different staining patterns. If the fixative used does not contain dichromate, a prestaining chromation step is usually adopted.

➤ **Is this procedure easy to carry out?**

The stain needs to be prepared in-house, and the time required for this varies between methods. Use of hematin gives a stain that may be used immediately, but has a short shelf-life. A PTAH solution prepared from chemically oxidized hematoxylin needs to stand for at least a day, with peak staining activity not being reached for a week.

However, the resulting stain has a longer shelf-life. Stain produced from air-oxidized hematoxylin does not reach its peak performance for several months; but can be used for several years.

All the variant PTAH stains are slow acting (12–24 h) at room temperature, although PTAH prepared directly from hematin is said to be the fastest acting. Staining can be achieved in only a few hours if carried out at 56°C, but this solution is considered to be less precise.

► Obtaining and keeping reliable reagents

1. Caution should be exercised when preparing PTAH directly from hematin, because commercial batches of hematin vary in dye content. Only use batches that look chocolate-brown as the dye paste is prepared, otherwise insufficient dye will be present to give a satisfactory staining solution.

2. For guidelines on the aging of the various PTAH preparations, see above.

3. For the methods using air oxidation, once sufficient aging of the stain has occurred, the solutions are stable indefinitely when stored at room temperature.

PROBLEMS AND HOW TO DEAL WITH THEM

► Tissue stains unexpectedly weakly

1. Insufficiently ripened PTAH solutions produce pale staining, so check with the above guidelines concerning reagent aging.

2. Stain can be lost during dehydration, so try a more rapid passage through the alcohols.

3. When staining astrocytes, if the glial fibrils are too pale, try treating with a mercuric fixative prior to staining.

4. Failure to use a prestaining oxidation step can result in overall pale coloration.

➤ **Staining is of an unexpected color**

1. If a section is too blue, try extending the period of dehydration, as this may provide a measure of selective removal.

➤ **Nature of staining is unusual**

1. If the pattern of staining is not as expected, did you use a heated staining procedure? If so, do not preheat the PTAH prior to staining. If this does not improve matters, try staining at room temperature.

2. If background deposits form excessively, try reducing the time in the dichromate fixative/mordant.

Background reading

A critical study of how practical variables influence PTAH staining patterns and reliability is available (Shum & Hon 1969). The chemistry of PTAH has been discussed (Bulmer 1962, Terner et al 1964); the chemistry of the heteropolyacids is concisely reviewed by Cotton & Wilkinson (1962: 786). The hematin content of commercial samples has been documented (Marshall & Horobin 1974b). The case for metachromasia is argued by Terner (1966), that for rate control by Bulmer (1962), and that for hydrogen bonding between stain and collagen by Puchtler et al (1980). An account of the influence of differential tissue permeability on the staining patterns of large and small acid dyes is given by Baker (1958).

43 Romanowsky–Giemsa stains

Background information

Romanowsky–Giemsa stains all contain the small, blue, cationic thiazine dye Azur B plus the large, red, anionic dye Eosin Y. Traditional Romanowsky–Giemsa stains are prepared from polychromed Methylene Blue and so are likely to contain additional thiazine dyes (e.g. Methylene Blue and several of its oxidation products).

Romanowsky–Giemsa methods are used to stain smears of blood, cytological preparations and microorganisms, and to band chromosome spreads. These stains are also occasionally used to stain histological tissue sections. Details of such procedures vary, but at some point they typically use neutral aqueous solutions containing Azur B and Eosin Y, stabilized by organic solvents such as methanol and glycerol.

Initial coloration involves acid and basic dyeing, with cationic Azur B staining anionic DNA and RNA blue, and anionic Eosin staining certain denser, polycationic protein-rich structures red. Subsequently, a purple Azur–Eosin complex or salt forms in chromatin and in neutrophil granules in blood, and in chromosomal G-bands. The mechanism by which the purple stain arises is disputed. However, it is agreed that the process is catalytic, with purple staining increasing continually with time of staining, without an equilibrium being reached. The purple material is only formed around neutral pH, and its formation is inhibited by excess organic solvent and by use of formalin fixation.

Staining intensity is particularly influenced by the concentration of Azur B, and by the Azur/Eosin ratio. The color balance of the staining is affected by a range of factors, such as the fixation, the pH and buffer salts of the working solution as well as the particular buffer salts used, the amount of organic solvent present, and the staining time.

See Plate 28.

Common variants

There are very many variants. However, until reasonably pure commercial Azur B became available in the 1980s none were standardizable, since the stain itself was so variable. There is no consensus on preferred color patterns; experienced personnel can make accurate diagnoses on specimens stained in all manner of ways.

AVOIDING PROBLEMS

➤ **What types of specimen processing are suitable?**

For most purposes specimens are fixed in methanol, although histological material fixed in Bouin's solution, formalin or Susa's solution can also be used. With smears, formaldehyde prevents the formation of the purple Azur–Eosin complex. Histological material can be embedded in paraffin or a hydrophilic resin.

➤ **Is this procedure easy to carry out?**

The methods are straightforward and, if standardized, are reliable with cell smears and chromosome spreads. Staining of histological materials is more variable, and modifications are required for paraffin or hydrophilic resin sections.

➤ **Obtaining and keeping reliable reagents**

1. Both Azur B and Eosin Y can now be obtained commer-

cially in reasonably pure form. If you propose preparing your own stock solutions, purchase such pure materials, checking both the dye content and the dye purity.

2. If you use commercial stock powders or solutions (e.g. labeled Giemsa's, Leishman's or Wright's stain), note that these are often manufactured from highly heterogeneous thiazine dyes, so standardization is not possible. Find a brand you like, and stick with it. Hopefully its composition will not change from one batch to another.

3. The stock solutions or powders are stable for long periods. To maximize shelf-life, store in cool, dark conditions, avoiding containers with metal caps.

4. Working solutions start to deteriorate as soon as they are made up, so discard working solutions that show substantial precipitation.

PROBLEMS AND HOW TO DEAL WITH THEM

➤ Stain or staining solution not as expected

1. Precipitates seen on slides can arise for several reasons:

    (a) The buffer concentration is too high. Check and adjust.

    (b) The methanol (or other organic solvent) content is too low. Check and adjust.

    (c) The staining solution is too old. Prepare a fresh working solution. In any event, abandon working solutions that show significant precipitation.

2. Stock solutions of Giemsa that have stood for a long time can still be used after agitation in an ultrasonic waterbath and remaking the working solution.

➤ Tissue stains unexpectedly weakly

1. Absence of staining of basophil granules can occur if the methanol used for fixation did not contain thiazine dye,

since granules are then not retained. Fix with methanol containing thiazine dye.

2. Weak staining of neutrophil granules occurs for various reasons:

   (a) The concentration of Azur B is too low. Use a standardized staining procedure, or try other batches of commercial stain. For additional possibilities see 'Leucocyte nuclei stain blue, not purple' below.

   (b) Even if there is sufficient Azur B present, purple granular staining will not occur if the Azur B/Eosin Y molar ratio diverges greatly from 8 : 1 to 10 : 1. Use a standardized staining procedure, or try other batches of commercial stain.

▶ Unexpected structures stain

1. 'Toxic granules' can arise in normal blood for several reasons:

   (a) The pH is above 8. Check and adjust.

   (b) The staining time is too long. Check and adjust.

   (c) The stain used has a higher Azur B content than you are used to.

▶ Staining is of an unexpected color

Leucocyte nuclei stain blue, not purple:

1. Azur B concentration is too low. This can have several causes:

   (a) The amount of Azur B is too low in the batch of stain used. Try another batch of commercial stain, or preferably use a standardized staining method.

   (b) In particular, stains prepared from dry powders low in Azur B become enriched in this crucial dye as air oxidation of the working solution takes place. Try leaving the working solution to stand for several days, or try another batch of commercial stain.

2. The Eosin has precipitated from the working solution. Check the amount of scum and, if this is appreciable, prepare a fresh working solution. Also see 'Stain or staining solution not as expected', above.

3. The pH of the working solution is too low. Check that it has not fallen below 5.5.

4. The staining time is too short. Try extending the time.

Lymphocyte cytoplasms are greyish-red, not blue:

1. The ratio of Azur B/Eosin Y is too low. Increase the ratio or use another batch of commercial stain.

2. In nonstandardized staining systems, the concentration of Methylene Blue may be too low, or the amounts of more highly demethylated thiazines are too high. Try another batch of commercial stain.

Eosinophil granules are brownish-orange rather than pink:

1. Some standardized stains always give this appearance. If you don't like this, rinse slides for 2 min in distilled water.

2. The stain is perhaps too alkaline, above pH 8. Check and adjust.

Eosinophil granules and erythrocytes are too blue:

1. The working solution is too alkaline, above pH 8. Check and adjust.

2. The staining time is too long. Check and adjust.

Background reading

For a review of hematological applications see Marshall (1980), of chromosome banding Bickmore & Sumner (1989), and of histological use Wittekind et al (1991). Mechanistic accounts include those by Wittekind & Gehring (1985) and Horobin & Walters (1987), which emphasize Azur–Eosin complex formation and staining-rate effects, respectively.

A typical standardized Romanowsky–Giemsa stain is that recommended by the International Committee for Standardization in Haematology (1984). Troubleshooting Romanowsky–Giemsa staining has been addressed explicitly by Horobin & Walters (1987) and Wittekind (1986: 34).

Individual staining procedures

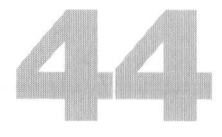

44 Rubeanic acid method for copper

Background information

Rubeanic acid (dithiooxamide) is a small compound, applied histochemically from a largely aqueous solution containing sodium acetate. Various counterstains are used (e.g. the basic dye Neutral Red or the acid dye Tartrazine).

Binding of the reagent to the tissues depends on the formation of an insoluble metal chelate with copper ions. Even in warm solutions this occurs slowly. Staining selectivity is partly a matter of copper giving a greenish-black chelate, whereas other metal ions give chelates of different colors. In addition, although formation of cobalt and nickel chelates may occur, these compounds are soluble in the presence of the sodium acetate, and so do not readily precipitate.

Rubeanic acid reacts only with free copper ions. Copper chelated by copper associated protein (CAP) must be released, by exposure to hydrogen chloride vapor, to permit its demonstration.

See Plate 29.

AVOIDING PROBLEMS

➤ **What types of specimen processing are useful?**

Neutral formalin is satisfactory as fixative, whilst fixatives containing metal ions, or which are acidic, must be avoided. Sections may be frozen, paraffin or celloidin.

➤ Is this procedure easy to carry out?

The method is simple and easy to carry out, although slow. Care must be taken to avoid metal ion contamination from water used in preparing the specimen and section, the stain and the rinses. Also, care must be taken to avoid such contamination from any reagents used, and indeed from the glassware.

➤ Obtaining and keeping reliable reagents

1. To avoid contamination by exogenous copper ions, use analytical-grade reagents and triple-distilled or de-ionized water.

2. Prepare the reagent freshly for each investigation.

➤ Useful routine control procedures

1. A section from a specimen known to contain copper should be stained, along with the experimental slide, as a positive control.

PROBLEMS AND HOW TO DEAL WITH THEM

➤ Tissue stains unexpectedly weakly

1. The copper chelate is formed very slowly, so try extending the staining time. (*Guideline*: Start at 16 h, and work up.)

2. If the copper is expected to be bound to CAP, then pre-treat a warmed section in hydrogen chloride vapor for 15 min before staining (Bancroft & Stevens 1996: 259).

➤ Unexpected structures stain

1. If excessive staining occurs, distributed randomly across the section, contamination by some external copper source may have occurred. Check if you used analytical-

grade reagents, multiply-distilled or de-ionized water, metal-free fixative and other reagents, and uncontaminated glassware.

➤ Staining is of an unexpected color

1. If the color of staining is blue-violet or yellowish-brown, perhaps cobalt or nickel ions are being demonstrated, not copper.

➤ Other problems

1. Sections are prone to lift from slides, due to the alkaline nature of sodium acetate. Use a section adhesive, and/or celloidinize the section before staining.

Background reading

The method was described by Uzman (1956).

45 Shikata Orcein method for hepatitis B antigen

Background information

Orcein is composed of a mixture of amino- and hydroxy-phenoxazone compounds. These result from the air oxidation of orcinol in the presence of ammonia. Some of these dyes, such as the amino orceins and amino orceimines, are cationic and possess large conjugated systems.

This method involves an initial oxidation of the section with an acid solution of permanganate. Manganese dioxide precipitated onto the section is bleached using oxalic acid. The oxidized section is then stained with a strongly acidic solution of Orcein, in aqueous alcohol. This gives a brown to black staining of the deposits of hepatitis B antigen in affected hepatocytes, as well as to certain additional structures.

The preliminary oxidation converts sulfur-containing proteins into sulfonic acids. Whilst most proteins contain some sulfur-containing amino acid residues, the sites of most significance in the present method are dense and/or sulfur-rich structures. The resulting sulfonate anions bind the cationic dye(s) present in the Orcein.

The extremely acidic character of the dye-bath inhibits staining of weaker tissue acids (e.g. carboxylated glycosaminoglycans, and phosphated DNA and RNA), since these will not be ionized, as does the substantially alcoholic solvent, since this does not permit hydrophobic bonding. In keeping with this mode of action, a variety of tissue sites do stain, and other basic dyes with large conjugated systems (e.g. Aldehyde Fuchsin and Alcian Blue) can replace the Orcein.

See Plate 30.

AVOIDING PROBLEMS

► What types of specimen processing are suitable?

This stain is applied to routine formalin-fixed, paraffin-embedded material.

► Is this procedure easy to carry out?

It is technically straightforward.

► Obtaining and keeping reliable reagents

Although commercial batches are still sometimes labeled 'natural', both commercial and natural Orceins are complex mixtures, and exhibit considerable batch variation. It has been suggested that modern Orcein is routinely synthetic. In the light of this, some tips may be offered:

1. When you use a fresh batch of Orcein, check its efficacy using a positive-control slide (see below). If this slide does not stain, try another batch of dye.

2. As an alternative, or if you have no positive-control slide, use a batch of Orcein the visible spectrum of which shows a distinct shoulder above 600 nm (for details see Iwamoto et al 1979).

3. The Orcein staining solution is not stable, prepare this freshly for each investigation.

► Useful routine control procedures

1. As a positive control for the efficacy of the method, stain a test section of material known to contain the antigen.

2. Retain a sample of a successful dye batch, and use this as a reagent control if doubtful staining occurs.

PROBLEMS AND HOW TO DEAL WITH THEM

▶ **Tissue stains unexpectedly weakly**

1. This can occur due to use of a poor batch of Orcein (see above).

2. Did you use freshly prepared Orcein? If not, try again with a fresh solution.

3. This is a slow procedure. Try staining for longer, checking under the staining microscope. (*Guideline*: 4 h in the Orcein solution at room temperature, 90 min at 37°C.)

▶ **Unexpected structures stain**

1. This method is not a specific stain, and various structures in addition to the antigen deposits may become colored. In particular, hepatocytes may contain CAP. Consider if the staining could be due to this.

Background reading

The original method was described by Shikata et al (1974). The chemistry of Orcein is concisely reviewed by Lillie (1977: 400). The role of the structure of Orcein, and of the acid alcoholic solvent, in enhancing the affinity and selectivity of Orcein constituents is discussed in a review by Horobin & Flemming (1980). For comments on the nature of commercial Orcein, see Green (1990: 544).

46 Solochrome Cyanine for myelin staining

Background information

The staining solution is prepared by reacting the anionic dye Solochrome Cyanine R with ferric ions, under strongly acid conditions. This results in the formation of three anionic metal complex dyes, one blue and two red, all of much the same size as the parent dye. If the pH of the staining solution is raised, a further anionic blue metal complex dye, which has an extremely large conjugated system, may be formed.

The staining procedure involves an initial nonselective overstaining with the acidic solution containing the metal complex dyes. Staining selectivity is achieved by a subsequent differentiation step, which removes stain from all tissue structures except myelin and erythrocytes, and, with some fixatives, nuclei.

The staining of myelin by Solochrome Cyanine may be regarded as involving an initial generalized acid dyeing of tissue protein by an anionic iron–dye complex(es). This is favored by the low pH (1.5) of the dye-bath, since this maximizes the number of tissue cationic groups. Staining selectivity arises in the subsequent de-staining step. This selectivity may reflect both the preferential retention of dye within dense, and so poorly permeable, structures, and/or the selective binding of basic groups present in myelin with the iron of the stain. Differentiators used differ in their mechanism of action. Some are alkaline, disrupting the acid dyeing; others are acidic solutions of ferric ions, which aid extraction of dye by formation of complexes of high iron/dye ratio in the differentiator solution.

Retention of the final stain in the tissues may be assisted by the in situ conversion of the dye(s) initially taken up into an iron complex dye with a large conjugated system, when the pH is raised during the final water washing. This larger dye would be able to form strong van der Waals attractions with the tissue proteins.

Common variants

There are variants of this procedure, but the differences between them do not seem profound. (*Note*: The synonym for Solochrome Cyanine R sometimes used in the histochemical literature is Chromoxane Cyanine R.)

AVOIDING PROBLEMS

➤ **What types of specimen processing are suitable?**

This method is applicable to cryosections or paraffin sections. Almost any fixative can be used, but the strongest and most selective coloration of myelin has been obtained after use of neutral formalin. If fixation is by Helly's, Susa or Zenker's fluids, the nuclear staining cannot be selectively removed by differentiation, and, although alcoholic fixatives permit staining, the myelin is not well preserved.

➤ **Is this procedure easy to carry out?**

This is a rapid and straightforward procedure. Even the differentiation is markedly easier than that in the alternative hematoxylin-based procedures.

➤ **Obtaining and keeping reliable reagents**

1. Satisfactory myelin staining may be obtained with Solochrome Cyanine samples the dye content of which is

within the range 35–55% of crude dye. Since the dye content of commercial batches of this dye have been reported to be around 45%, problems should not arise. However, assay and purification methods for Solochrome Cyanine R are available if needed (Kiernan 1984a).

2. Although iron alum can be used to generate the staining complex(es), this salt deteriorates on storage. Consequently, the appropriate concentrations of ferric chloride or ferric nitrate are preferable.

3. Sulfuric acid is as satisfactory as hydrochloric acid for preparing the staining solution.

4. Once prepared, the staining solution is stable, even in a clear bottle at room temperature, for years.

PROBLEMS AND HOW TO DEAL WITH THEM

➤ Tissue stains unexpectedly weakly

1. This can arise if the iron/dye ratio in the dye-bath is either too high or too low. First check your weighings. If you think these were correct, the dye content of the commercial Solochrome Cyanine could be too low or too high. Try another batch of dye, since most commercial dye samples seem satisfactory.

2. Overdifferentiation can very readily occur with the 'rapid' alkaline differentiators. Use shorter differentiation times or, if not experienced, make use of a 'slower' differentiator such as 5.6% aqueous ferric chloride solution.

3. Extraction of dye from the myelin into a counterstain can also occur if the counterstaining method involves an alkaline (pH > 8) or acidified alcoholic solvent. Avoid such counterstains.

➤ Unexpected structures stain

1. Blue staining of nuclei that cannot be selectively removed during differentiation can occur following the use of

fixatives such as Susa, Helly's and Zenker's fluids. If this feature is unacceptable, use a neutral formalin fixative in future work.

2. Blue nuclear staining can also arise if the iron/dye ratio in the dye-bath is too low. Check your weighings. If you think these were correct, try adjusting the molar iron/dye ratio a little, not to exceed 9.

Background reading

A critical and careful investigation of this type of procedure, and of the chemistry of the reagents involved, has been made by Kiernan (1984a, b).

47 Southgate's Mucicarmine stain for mucins

Background information

Southgate's Mucicarmine is prepared by heating Carmine, together with aluminum salts, in an acidic aqueous alcoholic solvent. Carmine is an ill-defined extract of cochineal insect, the active constituent of which is carminic acid, an anthraquinone species that carries glycoside, hydroxy and carboxylic acid substituents. The active species in staining is probably a cationic 2 : 1 carminic acid–aluminum chelate. This is a large dye, with a large conjugated system. Although one study found only a single dye in the staining solution, homogeneity could vary between batches, not least since carminic acid can lose its saccharide substituent on heating.

The Mucicarmine stain is applied following nuclear staining with an aluminum hematoxylin. Note that the staining solution contains a large excess of aluminum ions over that required to form any plausible aluminum–carminic acid complex, and the solvent is substantially alcoholic.

The likely mode of action of Mucicarmine is that the cationic metal complex dye binds to the anionic glycosaminoglycans present in mucins, in the usual basic dyeing mode. The selectivity, i.e. staining of mucins without displacing the counterstain from the nuclei, may be attributed to the large size of the dye, which is almost as large as the well-known mucin stain Alcian Blue. This results in a slow rate of dye diffusion, and hence restriction of staining to the permeable, and so fast staining, mucins.

Affinity will be enhanced by the large conjugated system, as indicated by the fact that stained sections can be dehydrated through the alcohols without loss. The odd staining patterns seen with certain mucins may be attributed to the presence of excess aluminum salts, inhibiting staining of some sites.

Common variants

There are related methods, including Mayer's Mucicarmine, of which Southgate's Mucicarmine was a modification, and Baker's Mucicarmine which some regard as superior, but others find very sensitive to variations in commercial Carmine.

AVOIDING PROBLEMS

➤ **What types of specimen processing are suitable?**

The method is routinely applied to formalin-fixed paraffin sections, but can be used with frozen sections, although images are then less clear.

➤ **Is this procedure easy to carry out?**

The stain has to be prepared in the laboratory, but may be stored in the refrigerator for 6 months or so. Once the stain has been prepared, the method is straightforward.

➤ **Obtaining and keeping reliable reagents**

1. Only some 20–40% of commercial Carmine is in the form of the staining component (i.e. carminic acid) present in accessible form. In practice, once you have obtained a good batch of Carmine, it is a valuable asset to the laboratory. Though it is possible to analyze commercial material for available carminic acid content, it is not worth the trouble. Try alternative suppliers, and only buy small amounts until you find a good supply.

2. Once the Mucicarmine has been prepared, the solution is stable in the refrigerator for about 6 months.

▶ **Useful routine control procedures**

1. With each batch of sections stained, add a section taken from a specimen known to contain mucins, as a positive control for the staining process.

PROBLEMS AND HOW TO DEAL WITH THEM

▶ **Tissue stains unexpectedly weakly**

1. Commercial samples of Carmine are variable in composition, so if weak staining occurs with a new batch of dye, purchase a new batch and prepare fresh Mucicarmine from that.

2. The stain deteriorates on standing, even in the refrigerator. Check the age of your working solution, and if it is more than a few months old prepare fresh Mucicarmine.

▶ **Unexpected structures stain**

1. If problems of this kind occur after use of a new batch of Carmine, purchase a new batch and prepare fresh Mucicarmine from that.

▶ **Staining is of an unexpected color**

1. If mucins look bluish, check that you did not use Ehrlich's hematoxylin as the nuclear counterstain, as this hematoxylin tends to stain some mucins. If Ehrlich's was not used, try extending the period of differentiation after the counterstain.

Background reading

For brief reviews of the chemistry of Carmine and its relationship to available carminic acid, see Green (1990:

190–192) and Marshall & Horobin (1974a). The latter authors also demonstrated the variability of commercial batches of Carmine. The chemistry of the putative 2:1 carminic acid–aluminum staining complex is discussed by Meloan et al (1971). The rate-control staining mechanism is discussed by Goldstein (1962).

48 Succinate dehydrogenase demonstration by an azodye method

Background information

The key reactants are succinate ion as substrate plus a tetrazolium salt as an electron acceptor/visualizing agent. The latter may be Nitro Blue Tetrazolium (NBT) or Tetranitro Blue Tetrazolium (TNBT), these being bistetrazolium salts with large conjugated systems. These both give rise to formazan reaction products that bind well to tissue proteins by van der Waals forces. Alternatively, methylthiazolyldiphenyl tetrazolium (MTT) may be used. The monoformazan which derives from MTT has a smaller conjugated system, with a lower substantivity. However, this may be transformed into a MTT formazan–cobalt chelate by treatment with cobalt ions. This chelate has a larger conjugated system, of higher substantivity.

Succinate dehydrogenase is the enzyme that catalyzes the dehydrogenation of succinate. When this occurs in the presence of a suitable tetrazolium salt the latter is reduced to an insoluble colored formazan.

See Plate 31.

Common variants

Three commonly used tetrazolium salts are MTT, NBT and TNBT. The former requires mounting in an aqueous medium, whilst the latter two can be dehydrated, cleared and mounted in a resinous medium.

AVOIDING PROBLEMS

➤ What types of specimen processing are suitable?

Fresh cryostat sections are used, with at most only a very brief fixation, or preferably a poststaining fixation.

➤ Is this procedure easy to carry out?

There are no particular problems with this procedure.

➤ Obtaining and keeping reliable reagents

1. Commercial samples of NBT or TNBT may be contaminated by significant amounts of the corresponding monotetrazolium salt, which gives rise to red staining rather than the expected blue coloration. If you wish to check monotetrazolium levels, use a thin layer chromatographic method (see Seidler 1991: 15). Alternatively, obtain another batch of reagent from a different supplier, since there is no easy way to remove such impurities.

2. Since MTT is relatively expensive, it is usual to freeze down aliquots of MTT incubation medium, in which form the salt is stable for several weeks.

➤ Useful routine control procedures

1. Omit substrate from the incubation medium. This will eliminate enzymic activity.

2. Alternatively, SDHase may be inhibited by 0.05 M malonate, if this is used both as a pretreatment and as an additive to the incubation medium.

PROBLEMS AND HOW TO DEAL WITH THEM

➤ Tissue stains unexpectedly weakly

1. The enzyme can be lost from fresh frozen sections. Add a

colloid-protecting agent, such as polyvinylpyrrolidone, to the incubation medium; alternatively, try fixing in acetone or formalin prior to staining.

2. However, since the enzyme is sensitive to formalin fixation, keep this brief.

3. If using MTT, the formazan of which is leached by non-aqueous mounting and mountants, check that an aqueous mountant was used.

▶ **Unexpected structures stain**

1. Direct reduction of tetrazolium salts is possible under alkaline conditions. Check that incubation was indeed carried out at the appropriate pH.

2. NBT can give rise to crystalline precipitates on the surfaces of fat droplets. Ignore this or, if this is a problem, try extracting the fat prior to staining using cold organic solvents.

▶ **Staining is of an unexpected color**

1. NBT can give rise to pink-purple staining, especially if the enzyme levels are low. This is either due to reduction to the half formazan, or to the presence of excessive contamination by the monotetrazolium salt (see above); the matter is disputed. In either event, this effect can be ignored, or you may remove the formazan from the sections by washing with acetone.

Background reading

Some of the biochemical aspects of these histochemical methods are discussed by Chayen & Bitensky (1991: especially 225–237).

49 Sucrase, by an azodye method

Background information

This is a simultaneous-coupling azodye method, the sections being incubated in a solution containing a naphthyl glucoside substrate and a diazonium salt visualizing agent. The substrate is 6-bromo-2-naphthyl-α-D-glucoside, the bromine substitution serving to increase hydrophobicity. The visualizing agent is Hexazotized Pararosanilin, which has a larger conjugated system than other diazonium salts commonly used in enzyme histochemistry.

During the incubation, a colorless bromonaphthol reaction product is formed from the glucoside by the action of sucrase. This naphthol is visualized by coupling with the diazonium salt, to form an azodye. Precise cellular localization of stain to the apical surface of the enterocytes, and resistance to extraction into solvents and mountants, is favored by the large conjugated system of the azodye, since this enhances dye–tissue protein binding.

AVOIDING PROBLEMS

➤ **What types of specimen processing are suitable?**

The method can be applied to unfixed cryostat sections, or to cryosections previously fixed in cold sucrose formalin. In any event, localization is enhanced by a poststaining fixation in formalin.

➤ Is this procedure easy to carry out?

The procedure is straightforward, although the diazonium salt must be freshly prepared by diazotizing pararosanilin with acidified nitrite immediately prior to use.

➤ Obtaining and keeping reliable reagents

1. It is necessary to prepare solutions of Hexazotized Pararosanilin freshly for each investigation. When doing this, you should ensure that sodium nitrite solutions used for diazotization are freshly prepared from recently opened containers.

2. The substrate solution is stable when stored frozen, and can be re-used a few times.

3. Do not overincubate, or crystal formation will occur.

➤ Useful routine control procedures

1. Staining should be totally prevented by enzyme inactivation (heat in boiling water for 10 min), or by omitting the substrate from the incubation solution.

2. Keep frozen sections of sucrase-positive specimens as positive controls.

3. Use a good positive control.

PROBLEMS AND HOW TO DEAL WITH THEM

➤ Stain or staining solution not as expected

1. When preparing the Hexazotized Pararosanilin the solution should go yellow soon after adding the sodium nitrite. If instead it goes brown or (at any subsequent point in the procedure) red, try another batch of pararosanilin, or a new bottle of sodium nitrite.

➤ Tissue stains unexpectedly weakly

1. To minimize extraction of the azodye reaction product into organic solvents, ensure that the passage through the

graded alcohols to xylene is rapid, and avoid contamination of alcohols by xylene.

➤ Unexpected structures stain

1. If the observed staining is general, rather than restricted to the apical edge of the enterocytes, try increasing the concentration of the Hexazotized Pararosanilin, but beware of enzyme inhibition.

2. Sulphated glycosaminoglycans (e.g. those in mucus goblet cells) may give false-positive staining due to binding of diazonium salts. This is nonenzymic, and so will be detected by using routine control procedure 1 (see above).

➤ Staining is of an unexpected color

1. Diazonium salts can react with tissue proteins. Thus with Hexazotized Pararosanilin yellow background staining can arise, especially if the pH rises above neutral. Check the pH of the incubation medium if this occurs.

Background reading

This method is described in the manual produced by Lojda et al (1979).

50 Sudan Black for lipids

Background information

Sudan Black is a nonionic, hydrophobic dye of moderate size. This dye can stain most lipids, and a generalized technical protocol follows. An optional prestaining bromination step may be used, which enhances staining of lipids, in particular of cholesterol, fatty acids and lecithin. Following this, an optional prestaining extraction with cold, anhydrous acetone will selectively remove hydrophobic lipids. Staining is then carried out using dye dissolved as a saturated solution in 70% aqueous ethanol. Any background staining is removed by differentiation with aqueous alcohol.

Such staining involves a partitioning process. Hydrophobic dye moves from the polar solvent into nonaqueous, lipid-containing regions of the specimen. The hydrated parts of the sections have only a low affinity for the dye, and any which does enter is removed by the differentiator. High-melting lipids, such as crystalline cholesterol deposits, will not stain unless brominated (bromination produces more hydrophobic and lower melting derivatives) or melted (as in the 'Burnt Sudan' method).

Sensitivity is strongly influenced by the solvent. Lipid can be extracted from the specimen during staining, and the polarity of the solvent controls partitioning. Moreover, since saturated solutions of Sudan Black are used, their concentration depends on the solvent's ability to dissolve dye.

Sensitivity is also influenced by access of stain to the lipid, with solid, and especially crystalline, lipids failing to stain. Hence the need for bromination, or elevated staining temperatures. Sensitivity is substantially influenced by the differentiation step and the polarity of the solvent.

Common variants

To increase dye concentrations, alternative solvents (e.g. propylene glycol, propanol and triethylphosphate) have been recommended. Suggested staining times range widely, from 1 to 30 min. To increase staining sensitivity, bromination pretreatment or heated staining procedures are needed.

AVOIDING PROBLEMS

➤ **What types of specimen processing are suitable?**

This method is usually applied to cryosections, since lipids are lost during paraffin embedding and de-waxing. With modifications, lipid in hydrophilic resin sections can be stained selectivity using Sudan Black, which provides superior morphological results (Gerrits et al 1992).

➤ **Is this procedure easy to carry out?**

This is a straightforward method.

➤ **Obtaining and keeping reliable reagents**

1. Commercial samples of Sudan Black routinely contain two black isomers plus smaller amounts of a number of other components.

2. Fresh dye solution is blue-black; on aging it becomes brownish-black. The time taken for this to occur varies, from days to weeks. Prepare a fresh solution at this stage, or play safe and replace stock solutions routinely each week.

➤ **Useful control procedures**

1. As a routine control, stain a section that has been de-

lipidized by extraction with chloroform–methanol. This solvent removes all lipids, so any Sudan Black staining will be artifactual.

2. To check whether Sudan Black staining is due to hydrophilic lipids (e.g. phospholipids), stain a section after extracting with cold, anhydrous acetone. This removes hydrophobic lipids, leaving the hydrophilic ones.

PROBLEMS AND HOW TO DEAL WITH THEM

➤ Stain or staining solution not as expected

1. Fresh dye solution is blue-black; on aging it becomes brownish-black. When this occurs, prepare a fresh dye solution.

➤ Tissue stains unexpectedly weakly

1. If the specimen is expected to be cholesterol-rich, staining is unlikely unless carried out following bromination, or at an elevated temperature. Use a prestaining bromination treatment or a 'Burnt Sudan' method.

2. If the method uses staining times in excess of 30 min, lipid may be extracted into the dye-bath. Try shorter staining times. If this does not help, try using a saturated solution of Sudan Black in 60% propanol or triethylphosphate for a shorter time.

➤ Unexpected structures stain

1. If nuclei or mucins stain, compare with a de-lipidized control. If such staining still occurs, the Sudan Black has probably decomposed, yielding basic products. Prepare a fresh batch of stain.

➤ Other problems

1. Aggregation of fat droplets into larger drops is encouraged both by bromination and the use of triethylphos-

phate as a solvent. If this is confusing, avoid such procedures.

Background reading

For background discussion of the method and its variants, and technical details of most of the procedures noted in this entry, see Bayliss High (1990).

51 Thiocholine cholinesterase method

Background information

This method requires acetylthiocholine as a substrate, with copper ions used as a trapping agent, and ammonium sulfide as visualizing agent.

The procedure demonstrates both acetylcholinesterase, as found in the nervous system and muscle, and also the cholinesterase present in several endocrine glands. These enzymes hydrolyze acetylthiocholine rapidly, liberating thiocholine. The latter is precipitated as colorless cuprous thiocholine iodide by reaction with copper and iodide ions, and this intermediate product transformed into brown copper sulfide by treatment with ammonium sulfide.

Should differentiation between the two enzymes be called for, then use of a duplicate section incubated in butyryl thiocholine demonstrates the cholinesterase specifically.

AVOIDING PROBLEMS

➤ **What types of specimen processing are suitable?**

Cryosections or vibratome preparations are suitable, and may be unfixed or fixed in acetone, formalin or glutaraldehyde (but see below).

➤ **Is this procedure easy to carry out?**

Preparation of the substrate solution requires centrifugation, with the use of the supernatant in the staining procedure.

➤ Useful routine control procedures

1. Incubate in substrate-free medium. This will totally prevent enzymic staining.

2. Both types of cholinesterase are inhibited by 0.3 mM physostigmine (eserine).

PROBLEMS AND HOW TO DEAL WITH THEM

➤ Tissue stains unexpectedly weakly

1. Cholinesterases are inhibited to some degree by formaldehyde, so if you fixed in formalin try using fresh cryostat sections.

2. Copper thiocholine may fail to precipitate in sites of low enzyme concentration. Try adding traces of copper thiocholine to the various fluids used in this procedure, to ensure that any that is formed enzymically will remain insoluble.

3. The sulfide ion content of the working ammonium sulfide solution decreases on standing, so make up fresh working solutions from stock each time.

➤ Unexpected structures stain

1. If particulate reaction product appears scattered randomly across the specimen, did you add copper choline to the wash water to limit reaction product loss? If so, make sure these solutions were free of suspended (i.e. insoluble) copper choline.

2. Are you sure the yellowish-brown coloration is due to reaction product? Beware endogenous pigments: use control procedure 1 (see above) to clarify this.

3. If the staining is diffuse around the enzymic site, try increasing the iodide content of the incubation medium,

since quantitative precipitation of the intermediate reaction product is dependent on the concentration of this ion. Alternatively, try adjusting the pH of the incubation medium.

4. If cell nuclei stain with enzymatically produced reaction product, this may be due to a diffusion artifact. Try adding sodium sulfate to the incubation medium; this often eliminates this problem.

5. Background staining is typically a light yellow. This is normal.

Background reading

A good account of the histochemical implications of the rather complex biochemistry of esterases is provided by Chayen & Bitensky (1991). The thiocholine procedures were critically investigated by Brzin and his collaborators; for a leading reference see Grubic & Brzin (1979).

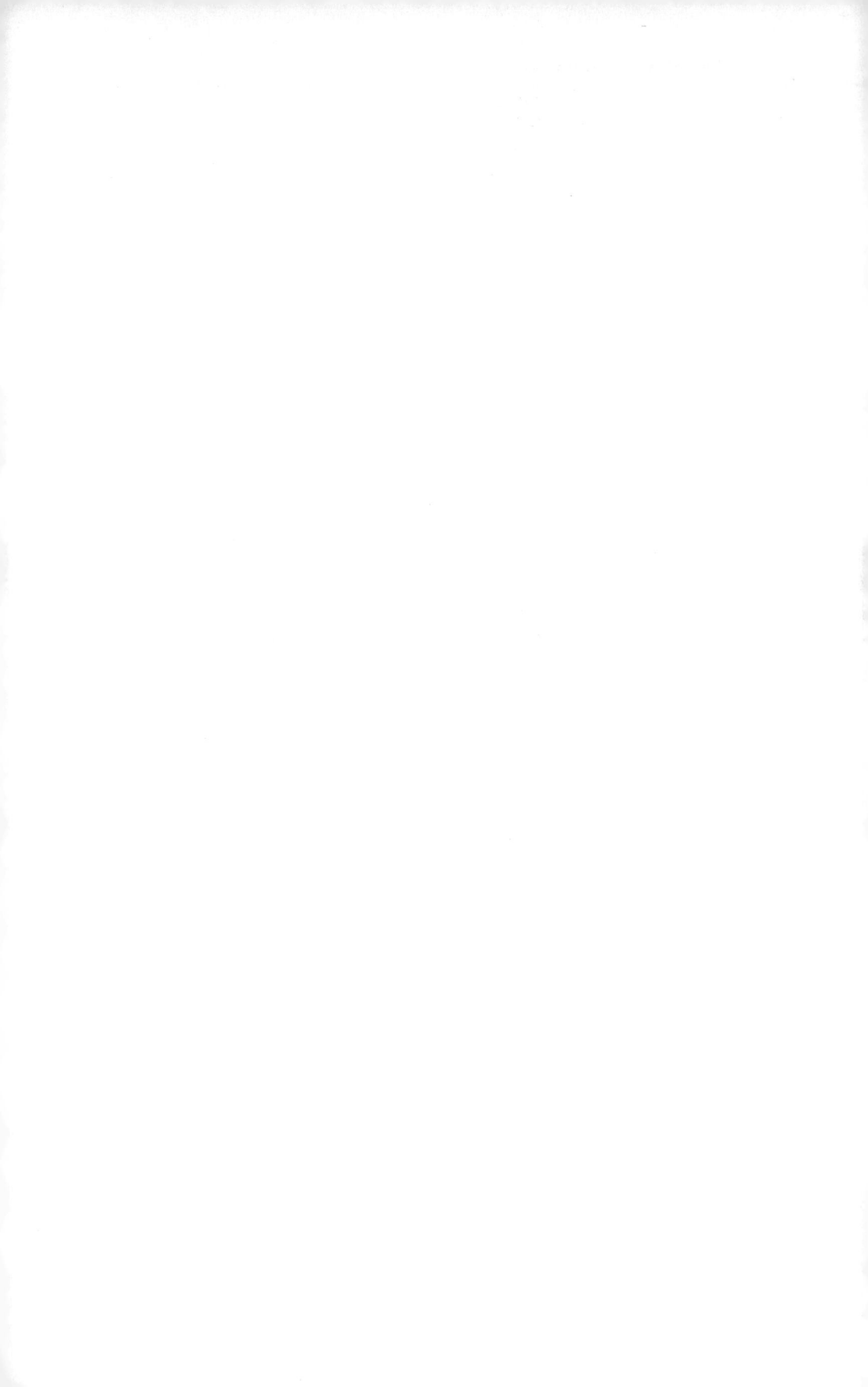

52 Thioflavine T method for amyloid

Background information

Thioflavine T is a small, highly fluorescent, cationic dye of moderate lipophilicity. In this procedure it is applied from aqueous solution, sometimes acidified strongly with hydrochloric acid or made salty with magnesium chloride. In any event, a poststaining acid differentiation is used to increase selectivity further.

Staining of amyloid is due to basic dyeing of anionic sulfated glycosaminoglycan or glycoprotein components of amyloid by the cationic dye. Van der Waals attractions may also contribute significantly to dye binding, facilitated by the high content of aromatic amino acids present in most amyloids. Whatever the precise mechanism, staining of amyloid is of higher affinity than that of other widely distributed basophilic sites, such as cell nuclei. In keeping with such a high affinity basic dyeing mechanism, selectivity is improved by lowering the pH of the dye-bath and by adding salt, both of which maneuvers inhibit basic dyeing. The same applies to the use of an acidic differentiator.

Common variants

The routine method applies the dye in water. Burn's variant uses dye dissolved in 0.1 M hydrochloric acid, to give greater selectivity.

AVOIDING PROBLEMS

➤ **What types of specimen preparation are suitable?**

Routinely, paraffin sections are used, and the mode of fixation is not critical. For research purposes cryosections may be used to give more sensitive staining. Whilst sections mounted in glycerol are the most intensely fluorescent, polystyrene mountants are usually satisfactory.

➤ **Is this procedure easy to carry out?**

The method is straightforward, without any significant complications.

➤ **Obtaining and keeping reliable reagents**

The dye solution is stable for several weeks or more, if stored in the dark.

➤ **Useful routine control procedures**

1. Look at unstained serial sections, to exclude confusion resulting from the presence of unusually strong autofluorescence.

2. Use sections freshly cut from amyloid-containing blocks as positive controls.

PROBLEMS AND HOW TO DEAL WITH THEM

➤ **Tissue stains unexpectedly weakly**

1. Check how the material was fixed. Staining of specimens fixed for several months in formalin is weak.

2. Check if the section has been left in daylight. Store in the dark, and preferably examine only recently stained sections. The staining is not light-fast.

➤ **Unexpected structures stain**

1. If the whole section stains strongly but nonselectively, check that you did indeed use Thioflavine T, and not

Thioflavine S, the latter being a chemically different dye with an unfortunately similar name.

2. If there is weak generalized fluorescence, check that Canada balsam was not used, since this mountant is itself fluorescent.

3. If basophilic structures stain nonselectively, check that the pH of the dye-bath and/or the differentiating solution is acidic, since lowering the pH suppresses much of the basophilia.

4. If nuclei fluoresce, check that you counterstained with Mayer's hematoxylin, which quenches nuclear fluorescence.

5. If arteriolar hyaline, elastic fibers, fibrinoid, the juxtaglomerular apparatus, keratin, mast cell granules, Paneth cells or zymogen granules fluoresce, ignore them. These structures typically stain by this method.

Background reading

The original method, still routinely used, was proposed by Vassar & Culling (1959). The most common modification, namely the use of a strongly acidic staining solution, was suggested by Burns et al (1967). The added-salt modification was devised by Mowry & Scott (1967). Investigations of the staining mechanism have been carried out by Burns et al (1967), Kelenyi (1967) and Mowry & Scott (1967), with some additional interesting observations being reported by Puchtler et al (1983).

53 Toluidine Blue for basophilia and metachromasia, and as an oversight stain

Background information

Toluidine Blue is a small, weakly hydrophilic cationic dye. When this dye is bound to DNA and RNA it is blue in color (orthochromatic). When bound to tissue constituents such as glycosaminoglycans, however, Toluidine Blue becomes reddish-purple, this spectral shift being termed 'metachromasia'.

There are numerous variant procedures, see below. However, the dye is typically applied as a dilute, weakly acidic, aqueous solution at room temperature. An important exception is the use of Toluidine Blue as an oversight stain for semi-thin epoxy-resin sections. In this case the dye is applied from a hot, alkaline dye-bath.

In all cases staining is basic dyeing. In slightly acidic solutions, the dye cations color tissue polyanions, including nucleic acids (DNA and RNA), which stain orthochromatically, and glycosaminoglycans (e.g. the heparin in mast-cell granules and the chrondroitin sulfate in cartilage matrix), which stain metachromatically red-purple. The reason for the purple color is that the dye ions are aggregated. This only occurs when bound to polyanions of high flexibility and charge density. Since hydrophobic bonding assists aggregation, metachromasia will be strongest in hydrated specimens, and will be inhibited by organic solvents.

In alkaline solutions, protein carboxyl groups are also ionized, so giving rise to a polychromatic staining of most tissue elements. In this case, staining patterns are strongly influenced by the presence of the resin, as reviewed by Horobin (1983). It is the resin that necessitates use of elevated staining temperatures, as penetration into these media does not occur at room temperature.

Sensitivity of staining thus depends on the pH of the working solution; and, in the staining of epoxy sections, on temperature. Occurrence of metachromasia is also influenced by the efficacy of poststaining dehydration, with strongest metachromatic staining being seen in wet-mounted sections, or in well-hydrated tissue structures, or both. Selectivity also depends on pH, and on the differentiation that occurs during dehydration.

See Plate 32.

Common variants

For cryosections and paraffin and hydrophilic resin sections dilute, acidic, aqueous solutions at room temperature are used. An exception is the concentrated, propanolic solution used for staining amyloid in paraffin sections. More concentrated alkaline aqueous solutions are used at elevated temperatures for epoxy sections.

AVOIDING PROBLEMS

➤ **What types of specimen processing are suitable?**

Variant methods can stain paraffin, cryogenic and hydrophilic resin sections; and also semi-thin epoxy resin sections. Fixation is not critical.

➤ **Is this procedure easy to carry out?**

These methods are easy to use and are usually straightforward. Staining of epoxy sections is likely to be the most variable, due to the hotplate heating method used.

➤ Obtaining and keeping reliable reagents

1. Commercial samples of Toluidine Blue usually contain de-methylated homologs as impurities. The dye content of such samples can, however, be high. Occasional samples are adulterated with other blue basic dyes, such as Thionin. However, even a chromatographically pure sample of Toluidine Blue gives metachromatic staining, including the green coloration of lignified plant materials. The presence of colored impurities is not usually significant.

2. Acidified aqueous solutions of Toluidine Blue are stable for long periods, but should be filtered before use.

3. Alkaline solutions stored at room temperature doubtless de-methylate, but nevertheless remain satisfactory for some months.

PROBLEMS AND HOW TO DEAL WITH THEM

➤ Tissue stains unexpectedly weakly

1. Toluidine blue is small, and hence fast diffusing, and is soluble in both water and ethanol. Consequently, dye is extracted into poststaining rinses, ethanolic dehydrating fluids and aqueous mountants. Blot, rather than rinse, in water after staining. Try using acetone or butanol rather than ethanol for dehydration, and beware aqueous mountants if permanent preparations are required.

2. Toluidine Blue fades. To delay this, store stained sections in the dark.

➤ Unexpected structures stain

1. If overstaining occurs, first try shortening the staining time.

2. However, if the background is strongly colored, or the staining time is already short, check the pH of the dye-bath. This, except for the epoxy sections, should be around pH 4. If necessary, add more acetic acid.

➤ **Staining is of an unexpected color**

1. If orthochromasia occurs, when metachromasia was expected, was the section overdehydrated? Is the mountant nonaqueous? View before dehydration, limit dehydration, or mount in an aqueous medium. Metachromasia is most intense in hydrated specimens.

Background reading

The easiest way to gather information on this group of methods is from a major manual. Two such books, which have good indexes, are those by Bancroft & Stevens (1996) and Lillie & Fulmer (1976). The influence of resin embedding media on staining patterns has been reviewed by Horobin (1983).

54 Van Gieson's and other picrotrichrome oversight and collagen stains

Background information

Van Gieson's Trichrome involves three dyes: yellow picric acid, which is small, anionic, and slightly hydrophobic; a red acid dye (e.g. Acid Fuchsin and Sirius Red), which is large and hydrophilic; and a metal complex cationic dye. This latter is usually either an iron hematoxylin or an iron Celestine Blue/aluminum hematoxylin sequence, although application of an aluminum hematoxylin is sometimes suggested.

Nuclei and basophilic cytoplasms are stained initially. The metal complex dyes recommended are usually selected to be stable in the subsequent acidic dye-bath. If necessary, staining is differentiated in acid alcohol. The second staining step involves an aqueous solution containing picric acid and the red acid dye, which gives a red coloration of collagen, with cytoplasms and other protein-rich material being stained in shades of yellow.

Van Gieson's staining involves acid and basic dyeing. Picric acid and the red acid dye are anions that stain proteins, since these are cationic at the low pH of usage. The cationic metal complex dyes stain DNA and RNA. The cause of differential staining by the two anionic dyes, with collagen fibers being selectively stained by red acid dye, is disputed.

One view regards staining patterns as rate controlled: the larger, slower diffusing, red acid dye only stains the most permeable sites, namely collagen fibers; whilst the smaller, faster diffusing picric acid reaches all acidophilic sites. A number of technical observations are congruent with this: fixatives that increase staining rates result in redder colorations, and thick sections stain yellower than thin sections. Nevertheless, recent work on the picro–Sirius Red method indicates that other, nonkinetic, factors play a significant role in that stain.

Selectivity is influenced by a variety of factors, including fixation, embedding media, section thickness, staining conditions (relative dye concentrations, pH and time), and rinse/dehydration conditions.

Common variants

Recommended dye concentrations, times, temperatures, and so on, vary. Closely related methods involve alternative small yellow dyes (e.g. flavianic acid or Naphthol Yellow S) and large red dyes (the traditional Acid Fuchsin, Sirius Red F3B or Violamine).

AVOIDING PROBLEMS

➤ **What types of specimen processing are suitable?**

With suitable, usually minor, modifications this procedure may be carried out with celloidin, cry-hydrophilic resin and paraffin sections. Although there are fixative effects on the color balance of staining, fixation is not critical.

➤ **Is this procedure easy to carry out?**

The method is straightforward.

➤ **Obtaining and keeping reliable reagents**

1. Commercial batches of picric acid are usually pure.

2. The red dyes usually recommended for this procedure are Acid Fuchsin and Sirius Red F3B. However, Acid

Fuchsin is routinely a mixture containing a variety of related dyes, and purchasers of 'Sirius Red' may plausibly acquire one of various related dyes. Fortunately, they will all work in the method, although they may not work as well.

3. If picro–Sirius Red solutions are stored, the red dye may eventually hydrolyze. Storing separate picric acid and Sirius Red solutions is recommended.

➤ Useful routine control procedures

1. Keep sections from a suitable 'well-staining' block for use as positive controls for stain and procedural efficacy.

PROBLEMS AND HOW TO DEAL WITH THEM

➤ Tissue stains unexpectedly weakly

1. Uneven staining of collagen fibers, with some areas of the sections being satisfactory, may be due to stain not being sufficiently acidic. Check the pH of the working solution.

2. If nuclei fail to stain, or are weakly colored, check that an iron hematoxylin or Celestine Blue was used. If an aluminum hematoxylin was used, replace with one of the aforementioned. In any event, ensure that nuclear staining is intense before application of the picro–red acid dye solution, since the picric acid acts as a differentiating agent.

➤ Unexpected structures stain

1. Noncollagenous structures (e.g. parotid gland secretion granules) may stain with Sirius Red. If such unusual staining occurs, check if a change in fixative has occurred, as such surprises may be fixative effects.

2. Staining of celloidin embedding media can occur if an iron Celestine Blue nuclear stain is used. Try using an iron hematoxylin nuclear stain.

▶ **Staining is of an unexpected color**

1. If sections are redder or yellower than you anticipate, check the fixative used. A coagulant fixative tends to produce redder tones, and a cross-linking fixative produces yellower colors.

2. With picro–Sirius variants, if red cytoplasmic staining occurs, check that you are preparing fresh working solution prior to staining. Sirius Red can eventually hydrolyze, especially under acid conditions and at higher temperatures, yielding small red dye products. If you work in a hot climate, beware.

3. If thick sections cut for neuroanatomical work are yellower than anticipated, this may be a section-thickness artifact. Try longer staining times, or staining in a heated dye-bath.

4. If sections become redder during removal of excess stain and dehydration, the small somewhat lipophilic picric acid may have been selectively extracted by the rinse (if used) or the dehydration alcohols, leaving an excess of the large hydrophilic red acid dye. Replace any aqueous rinse step by blotting, or rinsing in alcohol and/or shorten dehydration times.

5. Specimens embedded in hydrophilic resins may show no red staining in regions expected to be collagen-rich. This may be due to resin excluding the larger dye. Try longer staining times, adding a little ethanol to the staining bath as plasticizer, or staining in a heated dye-bath.

6. If sections become yellower on storage, the red acid dye may have faded. Acid Fuchsin is especially prone to do this. Keep out of direct sunlight.

▶ **Other problems**

1. If excessive wrinkling of hydrophilic resin-embedding media occurs, try increasing the amount of cross-linker in the resin mix (see Gerrits & Van Leeuwen 1987).

Background reading

The classic account of trichrome staining from a rate-control viewpoint is that by Baker (1958). A more recent demonstration of the importance of dye size can be found in a paper by Horobin & Flemming (1988), while a recent and extensive study emphasizing nonkinetic factors is given by Prento (1993). A paper oriented to troubleshooting trichromes is available (Shoobridge 1983).

55 Von Kossa technique for mineralized bone

Background information

This method involves the impregnation of the specimen in silver nitrate; with this being followed by application of an appropriate counterstain (e.g. Neutral Red or Safranin for nuclei, or Van Gieson's trichrome when the objective is to compare mineralized bone with unmineralized osteoid).

The silver impregnation is achieved using an aqueous silver nitrate solution. When staining sections, this is carried out in bright sunlight or under strong artificial illumination. Excess unreduced silver nitrate is removed using thiosulfate, and an appropriate counterstain applied. When specimens are impregnated in the block, this is done in the dark, and the silver subsequently reduced chemically with hydroquinone or an equivalent agent.

Mechanistically, the first step is the ion exchange of tissue calcium ions with the silver cations. Once bound to the tissue in this way, as poorly soluble silver phosphate and carbonate, the cations may be reduced chemically to metallic silver microcrystals, this being essential with block impregnation. With impregnated sections, reduction is usually achieved by using strong illumination, the actual reducing agent being organic constituents of the tissue section.

In this latter type of procedure, unreduced silver cations are then removed in a water wash, following their conversion to complex anions of high water solubility by treatment with thiosulfate. Counterstaining involves acid or basic dyeing, with appropriate dyes.

See Plate 33.

Common variants

This procedure may be carried out on sections cut from tissue blocks containing mineralized material. When the amount of mineralization would make this impracticable, the tissue blocks may be silver stained, then decalcified and prepared for sectioning.

Routinely, the silver cations in sections are photoreduced to metallic silver, whereas after block impregnation reduction is achieved by a chemical reagent such as hydroquinone.

AVOIDING PROBLEMS

➤ **What types of specimen processing are suitable?**

This procedure is usually applied to tissue fixed in neutral buffered formalin, avoiding acidic fixatives, or formulations containing calcium salts. To obtain maximum sensitivity, alcoholic fixatives have been recommended. Paraffin sections are used.

➤ **Is this procedure easy to carry out?**

With the section procedure, staining is carried out under microscopic control.

PROBLEMS AND HOW TO DEAL WITH THEM

➤ **Tissue stains unexpectedly weakly**

1. Deposits of calcium salts may be lost prior to staining if the specimen is exposed to acids. Avoid acidic fixatives. Indeed, to maximize the retention of calcium salts, use alcoholic fixatives.

2. If mineralized bone is slow to blacken, check the illumination procedure. The use of a quartz halogen micro-

scope lamp is recommended, since a tungsten lamp emits less ultraviolet radiation and is less effective. Sunlight is, of course, ultraviolet-rich, but we write in England, where this natural resource may not be as reliably available as in other parts of the world.

➤ **Unexpected structures stain**

1. This is not a specific stain, and melanin also tends to blacken.

➤ **Nature of staining is unusual**

1. Granular background staining is more likely with chemical reduction, so if such deposits occur when staining sections, use the light-activated procedure.

➤ **Other problems**

1. When sections are cut from mineralized specimens, which tear during microtomy, celloidinize the sections before staining. Or, if necessary, carry out the silver impregnation in the dark, then decalcify and process through to paraffin.

2. The formation of black deposits, on the slide or section, may be triggered by contaminated glassware or the use of metallic instruments. Clean all glassware scrupulously, and avoid using such implements as metal forceps.

Background reading

The original Von Kossa method was described in 1901. A widely used block-impregnation variant is that of Trip & Mackay (1972). The most extensive scientific investigations of silver staining are those done by Gallyas (see, in particular, Gallyas 1979, 1982).

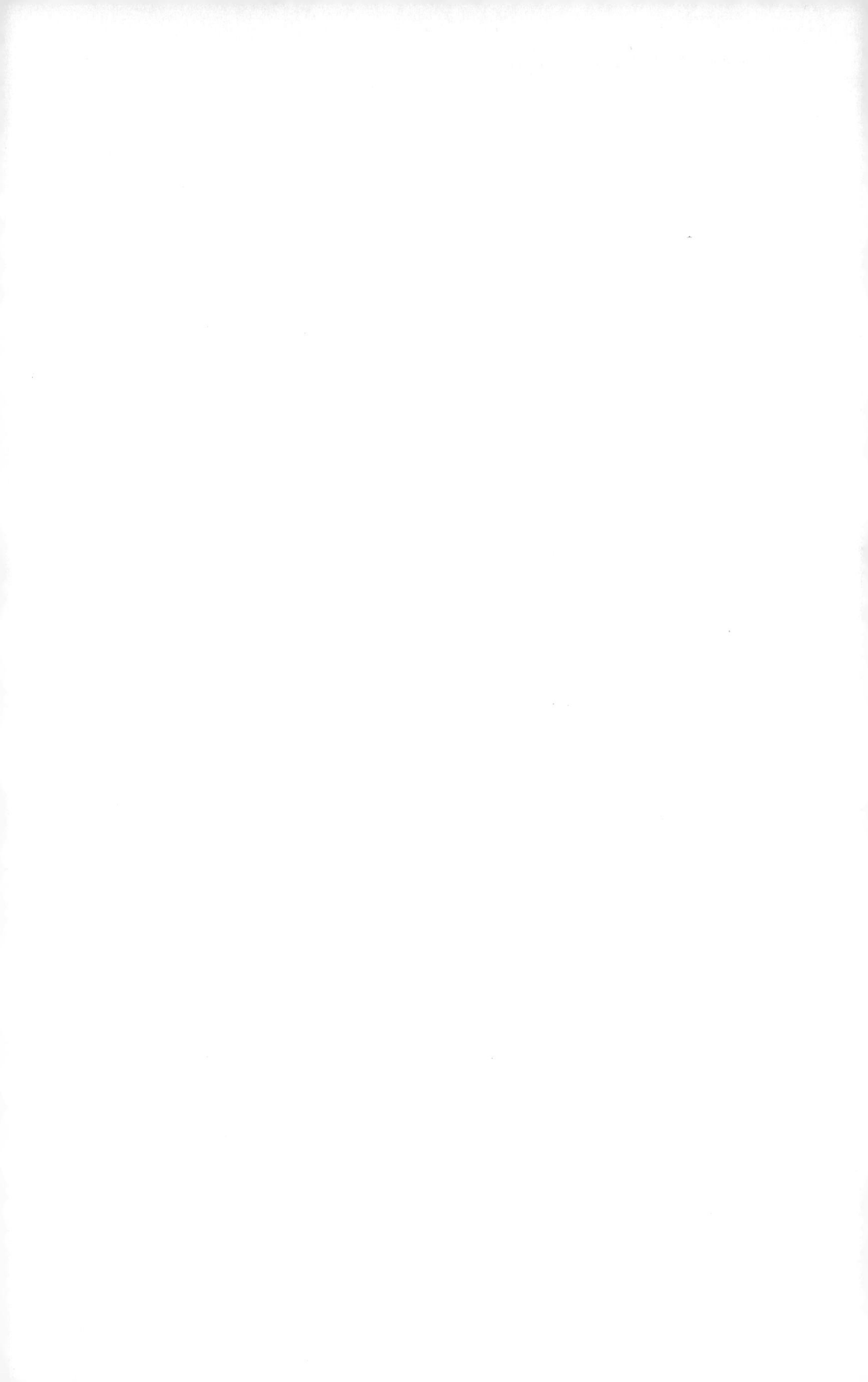

Individual staining procedures

56 Warthin–Starry method for spirochetes

Background information

This is a silver stain, the metal impregnation step of which uses silver nitrate. Development is achieved using a solution containing silver nitrate, hydroquinone and gelatin. Gold chloride is used for intensification.

Crucial staining steps are: impregnation in hot, aqueous acidic silver nitrate; development in a hot mixture of hydroquinone, silver nitrate and gelatin; and subsequent intensification using gold toning, if desired.

The staining mechanism is complex, and uses a physical developer. An initial impregnation in acidic silver nitrate results in the formation of microcrystals of metallic silver due to the reduction of silver cations, especially in the spirochetes. These microcrystals subsequently act as catalytic sites where silver cations, diffusing from the developer, are reduced by the hydroquinone to generate the larger crystals of metallic silver responsible for the visible staining. The gold toning deposits gold at the site of the silver, again catalyzed by the silver crystals.

See Plate 34.

Common variants

A number of variants of the original procedure have been

described (e.g. those of Bridges and Luna and of Faulkner and Lillie).

AVOIDING PROBLEMS

➤ What types of specimen processing are suitable?

The procedure is routinely carried out with formalin-fixed paraffin sections. Other fixatives can be used, but reagents containing heavy metals must be avoided.

➤ Is this procedure easy to carry out?

This is a rather time-consuming procedure. The method calls for some expertise, since the degree of contrast achievable between spirochetes and tissue background is not high.

➤ Obtaining and keeping reliable reagents

1. It is important that the developer constituents are mixed immediately prior to use.

2. Do not use old solutions, or use working solutions more than once.

➤ Useful routine control procedures

1. Use a section from a specimen known to contain spirochetes as a positive control.

PROBLEMS AND HOW TO DEAL WITH THEM

➤ Tissue stains unexpectedly weakly

1. If the spirochetes are weakly stained, increase the time in the developer. (*Guideline*: On first runs, use a series of developing times such as 3, 6, 8 and 12 min. Check the positive controls to see which time gives the most contrast staining.) If even long development times are ineffectual, increase the silver impregnation time.

➤ Unexpected structures stain

1. If the background staining is too strong, check that the

fixative used did not contain heavy metals, which must be avoided.

2. If the fixative was heavy-metal free, decrease the time in the developer. (*Guideline*: On first runs, use a series of developing times such as 3, 6, 8 and 12 min. Check the positive controls to see which time gives the most contrasty staining.) If even short times give overstaining, decrease the silver impregnation time.

3. Background staining also rises as the developer ages; check this, and if necessary replace with fresh solution.

4. This method is not specific for spirochetes. Other common organisms, and tissue materials such as melanin, will also stain black.

5. Check that stained organisms are within, not on, the surface of the section. If the latter phenomenon does occur, check that you used fresh distilled water for floating out the sections, so avoiding such microbial contamination.

➤ Nature of staining is unusual

1. If background staining takes the form of a precipitate, and is heavy, check that the section has been celloidinized and that the temperature of the silver impregnation solution was not too high.

➤ Other problems

1. Contaminants can trigger reduction of silver, so if the slide becomes covered with silver, clean the glassware scrupulously, and also use plastic, not metal, forceps.

Background reading

The original method was described by Warthin & Starry (1920). Some discussion of permissible variations has been provided by Bridges & Luna (1957) and by Faulkner & Lillie (1945).

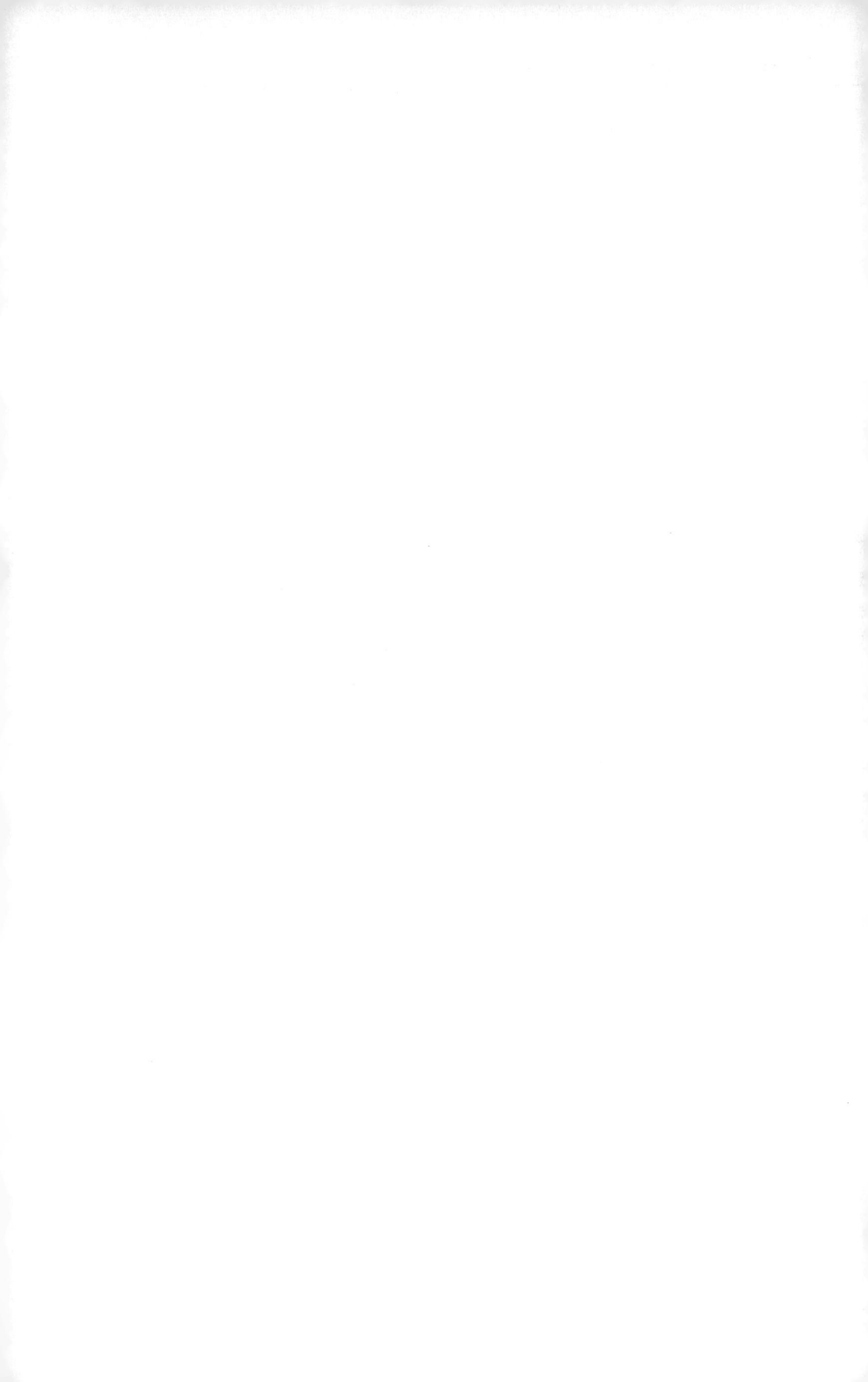

57 Ziehl–Neelsen and related stains of acid-fast bacteria

Background information

The primary stain in all Ziehl–Neelsen (ZN) variants usually contains Basic Fuchsin or one of its constituents (e.g. pararosanilin or New Fuchsin), although Victoria Blue R or Night Blue have sometimes been substituted. Following a red primary dye, the counterstain is usually Methylene Blue, or occasionally some other blue or green cationic dye (e.g. aluminum hematoxylin, Janus Green or Malachite Green). A red counterstain (e.g. Safranin) is applied following a blue primary dye. Cationic dyes used in the ZN methods all have conjugated systems of moderate size. Both the primary dye and the counterstain can vary from hydrophilic (pararosanilin and aluminum hematoxylin) to lipophilic (Victoria Blue and Malachite Green).

The primary staining solution also contains a cosolute. This is traditionally phenol, although anionic surfactants (e.g. Teepol or Tween) can be substituted; aniline, and other phenolic compounds, have also been used.

Whichever ZN procedure is used, certain key steps are required. First, the specimens are stained with Basic Fuchsin, or a substitute. This step is nonselective, and both mycobacteria and the tissue background are stained. Often this involves a hot dye-bath containing phenol or a substitute. The specimen is then differentiated in acid alcohol, until only the mycobacteria retain the primary dye. Subsequently, the specimen is counterstained with the other basic dye.

The mechanism of the ZN stain can be described as follows. The affinity of the primary dye for mycobacteria is due to basic dyeing of the various anionic materials found within these cells: DNA and ribosomal RNA, as well as membrane constituents such as mycollic acids and sulfated polysaccharides. Staining selectivity depends on the differentiation step. This selectivity is due to mycobacteria being particularly impermeable objects, resulting in slow dye diffusion, and hence slow dye loss from stained bacterial cells. Note that nonmycobacterial entities that stain (e.g. hair shafts, red blood cells and spermatozoa heads) are dense, and so impermeable.

The role of phenol and the use of an elevated staining temperature in the primary staining process is to increase the amount of dye in solution, and hence to increase the rate of staining of the poorly permeable, slow-staining, mycobacteria. The wide range of cosolutes that have been reported as effective (e.g. aniline, surfactants and phenols) is consistent with this view. As are the observations that low staining temperatures or omission of cosolutes can give rise to a standard staining picture if extended staining times are used. The counterstain colors cell nuclei, and in variants using alkaline solutions (e.g. Loeffer's Methylene Blue), protein-rich cytoplasms also, both by routine basic dyeing processes.

See Plate 35.

Common variants

As noted above, various primary dyes, various cosolutes and various counterstains can be used. Elevated staining temperatures can be avoided if staining times are extended; the same holds for the presence of phenol in the primary staining solution.

AVOIDING PROBLEMS

➤ What types of specimen processing are suitable?

The ZN method can be carried out on specimens fixed in formalin or most other fluids, except Carnoy's. Paraffin or cryosections may be used.

➤ Is this procedure easy to carry out?

If hot staining is used, it is safer and more reproducible to carry this out in a Coplin jar placed in a waterbath. The timing of the differentiation step is not critical, since it is hard to overdifferentiate.

➤ Obtaining and keeping reliable reagents

1. Carbol Fuchsin solutions are typically stable for months or even years.

2. Check how much of the dark-red deposit, precipitated during storage, does not redissolve on heating. If this is significant, prepare a fresh batch of stain.

➤ Useful routine control procedures

1. Keep a specimen containing mycobacteria, and take sections from this through the staining procedure, as a positive control.

PROBLEMS AND HOW TO DEAL WITH THEM

➤ Stain or staining solution not as expected

1. When using a ZN method based on Carbol Fuchsin, has this stain deposited substantial amounts of red precipitate? If so, discard and prepare fresh stain.

➤ Bacteria stain unexpectedly weakly

1. Compare with the positive control (see above), and if this is also weak check if the stain has been freshly prepared.

2. Exposure of the specimen to acids can reduce or eliminate acid fastness. So:

   (a) Check if an acidic fixative (e.g. Carnoy's fluid) has been used. If so, avoid this in future.

   (b) Check if the specimen has been decalcified in strong acid media. If so, use an alternative decalcification system in future.

3. If a Carbol Fuchsin stain was used, has this stain deposited substantial amounts of red precipitate? If so, discard and prepare fresh stain.

4. If a 'cold' method was used, the specimen might be understained. Extend the staining period (try overnight).

5. Are there few or no stainable organisms, even though the histological characteristics are indicative of tuberculosis? If so, check if the patient had been treated with routine antituberculous drugs, since these can result in nonstaining organisms.

6. If counterstaining is too intense, it can obscure the mycobacteria. If this appears likely, try counterstaining for a shorter time, or from an acidified solution.

▶ **Unexpected structures stain**

1. Does differentiation fail to remove background staining by the primary dye? Differentiation is slower with thicker specimens, so check the thickness. In any event, with existing specimens extend the time in the acid differentiator; be relaxed about this, it is difficult to overdifferentiate. Alternatively, try a method using a surfactant as cosolute, rather than phenol; or try a 'cold' method, which avoids heating the Fuchsin solution.

2. Does the counterstain give excessive coloration of the background? If so, counterstain for a shorter time, or counterstain from an acidified dye-bath.

➤ **Nature of staining is unusual**

1. Check that stained bacteria are in the focal plane of the section. If not, these acid-fast bacteria may be contaminants from the water supply.

2. If you stain by heating individual slides, and there are darkly stained 'odd-shaped' objects present, try staining in a Coplin jar in a heated waterbath. Dye can precipitate if the solution is overheated, causing excessive evaporation.

Background reading

Obviously, vast numbers of papers record the use of this method. Moreover, work has been done on the procedure's physicochemical basis. However, to the authors' surprise, there appears to be no critical extended review of this classic stain. The reader seeking wisdom can, however, start with Clark (1973: 250).

58 Ziehl–Neelsen technique modified for leprosy bacilli

Background information

The primary stain contains the cationic dye Basic Fuchsin, or one of its constituents (e.g. New Fuchsin), plus phenol as a cosolute (i.e. Carbol Fuchsin). The counterstain is usually the cationic dye Methylene Blue, or some acid dye/basic dye staining system such as hematoxylin and Eosin.

This procedure can be thought of as a modified Ziehl–Neelsen (ZN) technique. All the modifications reflect the fact that Carbol Fuchsin-stained leprosy bacilli are much less acid- and alcohol-fast than ZN-stained tubercle bacilli. The first modification is the use of a mixture of xylene and a vegetable oil for de-waxing the sections. Clove, cottonseed, groundnut (i.e. peanut), olive and origanum oils have all been recommended for this purpose. The second modification of the ZN method is to avoid alcohol dehydration during de-waxing. The sections are stained in Carbol Fuchsin at room temperature. This is followed by a differentiation in an acidic solution; both acid alcohol and aqueous sulfuric acid have been recommended. Counterstaining is with Methylene Blue, or some other tissue stain such as hematoxylin and Eosin. A final modification of the routine ZN procedure is that, following staining, alcohol dehydration is avoided, and sections are air dried.

Some plausible suggestions as to the mode of action of this stain may be offered. Affinity of the primary dye for leprosy bacilli is due to basic dyeing of the various anionic materials found within these cells; in particular, DNA and ribosomal RNA. Staining selectivity depends on the differentiation step. This selectivity is due to leprosy bacteria being relatively impermeable objects, resulting in slow dye diffusion, and hence slow dye loss from stained bacterial cells. Note that nonmycobacterial entities that stain by this method (e.g. hair shafts and, to a lesser extent, red blood cells) are dense, and so impermeable. The role of phenol in the primary staining process is probably to increase the amount of dye in solution, and hence to increase the rate of staining of the poorly permeable, slow-staining, leprosy bacteria. The counterstain colors cell nuclei, and in variants using an acid dye, cytoplasms by routine basic and acid dyeing processes.

See Plate 36.

Common variants

The modified ZN methods typically follow the suggestions of Fite et al (1947). However, Fite (1940) also suggested further modifications (e.g. a post-primary-stain formalin treatment), and later workers have combined and renamed these possibilities in a somewhat confusing way.

AVOIDING PROBLEMS

➤ **What types of specimen processing are suitable?**

This method is routinely applied to formalin-fixed paraffin sections.

➤ **Is this procedure easy to carry out?**

This method is straightforward to perform.

➤ **Obtaining and keeping reliable reagents**

Carbol Fuchsin solutions are typically stable for months or even years.

▶ Useful routine control procedure

1. Keep a specimen containing leprosy bacilli, and take sections from this throughout the staining procedure, as a positive control.

PROBLEMS AND HOW TO DEAL WITH THEM

▶ Tissue stains unexpectedly weakly

1. Exposure of the specimen to acids can reduce or eliminate acid fastness. So:

   (a) Check if an acidic fixative (e.g. Carnoy's fluid) has been used. If so, avoid this in future.

   (b) Check if the specimen has been decalcified in strong acid media. If so, use an alternative decalcification system in future.

▶ Unexpected structures stain

1. Does differentiation fail to remove background staining by the primary dye? Differentiation is slower with thicker specimens, so check the thickness.

2. This method is not specific for leprosy bacteria. For example, other acid-fast bacteria, and also tissue constituents such as hair shafts and even erythrocytes, stain.

▶ Staining is of an unexpected color

1. Does the counterstain give excessive coloration of the background? If so, make sure you use weak solutions of such counterstains as Methylene Blue. Alternatively, use shorter periods of counterstaining.

▶ Nature of staining is unusual

1. Check that stained bacteria are in the focal plane of the section. If not, these acid-fast bacteria may be contaminants from the water supply.

Background reading

The original Fite 'oil de-waxing' modification is described in Fite et al (1947). For the poststaining formalin treatment, see Fite (1940).

References

Andersson G K A, Kjellstrand P T T 1975 A study of DNA depolymerisation during Feulgen acid hydrolysis. Histochemistry 43: 123

Bach P H, Baker J R J (eds) 1991 Histochemical and immunohistochemical techniques. Chapman & Hall, London

Baker J R 1958 Principles of biological microtechnique: a study of fixation and dyeing. Methuen, London

Baker J R 1962 Experiments on the action of mordants. 2. Aluminium hematein. Quarterly Journal of Microscopical Science 103: 493

Bancroft J D, Cook H C 1994 Manual of histological techniques and their diagnostic application. Churchill Livingstone, Edinburgh

Bancroft J D, Stevens A (eds) 1990 Theory and practice of histological techniques, 3rd edn. Churchill Livingstone, Edinburgh

Bancroft J D, Stevens A (eds) 1996 Theory and practice of histological techniques, 4th edn. Churchill Livingstone, New York

Bartholamew J W 1962 Variables influencing results, and the precise definition of steps in Gram staining as a means of standardising the results obtained. Stain Technology 37: 139

Bartholamew J W, Mittwer T 1950 The mechanism of the Gram stain. II. The function of iodine in the Gram stain. Stain Technology 25: 169

Bartholamew J W, Mittwer T 1951 The mechanism of the Gram stain. III. Solubilities of dye-iodine precipitates and further studies of primary dye substitutes. Stain Technology 26: 231

Bayliss High O B 1990 Lipids. In: Bancroft J D, Stevens A (eds) Theory and practice of histological techniques, 3rd edn. Churchill Livingstone, Edinburgh, p 215

References

Bennion P J, Horobin R W 1974 Some effects of salts on staining: use of the Donnan equilibrium to describe staining of tissue sections with acid and basic dyes. Histochemistry 39: 71

Bettinger C H, Zimmermann 1991 New investigations on hematoxylin, hematein, and hemateinaluminium complexes. 2. Hematein–aluminium complexes and hemalum staining. Histochemistry 96: 215

Bickmore W A, Sumner A T 1989 Mammalian chromosome banding – an expression of genome organisation. Trends in Genetics 5: 144

Boon M E, Druijver J S 1986 Routine cytological staining techniques. Macmillan, London

Boon M E, Kok L P (eds) 1986 Standardisation and quantitation of diagnostic staining in cytology. Coulomb Press, Leiden

Bridges C H, Luna L 1957 Kerr's improved Warthin–Starry technique. Study of the permissible variations. Laboratory Investigation 6: 357

Brooke M H, Kaiser K K 1974 The use and misuse of muscle histochemistry. Annals of the New York Academy of Science 228: 121

Bulmer D 1962 Observations on histological methods involving the use of phosphotungstic and phosphomolybdic acids, with particular reference to staining with phosphotungstic acid/hematoxylin. Quarterly Journal of Microscopical Science 103: 311

Burns J, Pennock C A, Stoward P J 1967 The specificity of staining of amyloid deposits with Thioflavine T. Journal of Pathology and Bacteriology 94: 337–344

Butterworth P J 1983 Biochemistry of mammalian alkaline phosphatases. Cell Biochemistry and Function 1: 66

Chayen J 1968 The histochemistry of phospholipids and its significance in the interpretation of the structure of cells. In: McGee-Russell S M, Ross K F A (eds) Cell structure and its interpretation. Arnold, London

Chayen J, Bitensky L 1991 Practical histochemistry, 2nd edn. Wiley, Chichester

Chung C F, Chen C M C 1970 Restoring exhausted Schiff reagent. Stain Technology 45: 91

Clark G 1973 Staining procedures used by the Biological Stain Commission, 3rd edn. Williams & Wilkins, Baltimore

Clark G 1979 Displacement. Stain Technology 54: 111

Clasen R, Simon R G, Scott R, Pandolfi S, Laing I, Lesak A 1973 The staining of the myelin sheath by Luxol dye techniques. Journal of Neuropathology and Experimental Neurology 32: 271

Cooper J D, Payne J N, Horobin R W 1988 Accurate counting of neurons in frozen sections: some necessary precautions. Journal of Anatomy 157: 13

Cotton A, Wilkinson G 1962 Advanced inorganic chemistry. Interscience, London

Demalsy P, Callebaut M 1967 Plain water as a rinsing agent preferable to sulfurous acid after the Feulgen nucleal reaction. Stain Technology 42: 133

Dubowitz V 1985 Muscle biopsy, a practical approach. Baillière Tindall, London

Dunnigan M G 1968a Chromatographic separation and photometric analysis of the components of Nile Blue sulphate. Stain Technology 43: 243

Dunnigan M G 1968b The use of Nile Blue sulphate in the histochemical identification of phospholipids. Stain Technology 43: 249

Elleder M, Lojda Z 1970 Studies in lipid histochemistry. 2. The nature of the material stained with acid hematein test and with ORAN reactives in red blood cells. Histochemie 24: 21

Faulkner R R, Lillie R D 1945 A buffer modification of the Warthin–Starry silver method for spirochaetes in single paraffin sections. Stain Technology 20: 81

Filipe M I, Lake B D (eds) 1990 Histochemistry in pathology, 2nd edn. Churchill Livingstone, Edinburgh

Fishbein W N, Armrustmacher V W, Griffin J L 1978 Myoadenylate deaminase defficiency – a new disease of muscle. Science 200: 545

Fite G L 1940 The Fuchsin–formaldehyde method of staining acid-fast bacilli in paraffin sections. Journal of Laboratory and Clinical Medicine 25: 743

Fite G L, Cambre P J, Turner M H 1947 Procedure for demonstrating lepra bacilli in paraffin sections. Archives of Pathology 43: 624

Galassi L 1993 A simple procedure for crystallization of the Schiff reagent. Biotechnic and Histochemistry 68: 175

Gallyas F 1979 Factors affecting the formation of metallic silver and the binding of silver ions by tissue components. Histochemistry 64: 97

Gallyas F 1982 Physico-chemical mechanism of the argyrophil I reaction. Histochemistry 74: 393

Gerrits P O, Van Leeuwen M B M 1987 Glycol methacrylate embedding in histotechnology: the hematoxylin–eosin stain as a method for assessing the stability of glycol methacrylate sections. Stain Technology 63: 181

Gerrits P O, Horobin R W, Wright D 1990 Staining sections of

References

water-miscible resins. 1. Effects of the molecular size of the stain, and of resin cross-linking, on the staining of glycol methacrylate embedded tissues. Journal of Microscopy 160: 279

Gerrits P O, Brekelmans-Bartels M, Mast L, s'-Graavenmade E J, Horobin R W, Holstege G 1992 Staining myelin and myelin-like degradation products in the spinal cords of chronic experimental allergic encephalomyelitis (Cr-EAE) rats using Sudan Black B staining of glycol methacrylate-embedded materials. Journal of Neuroscience Methods 45: 99

Gimenez D F 1964 Staining Rickettsiae in yolk sac cultures. Stain Technology 39: 135

Goldstein D J 1961 Correlation of size of dye particle and density of substrate, with special reference to mucin staining. Stain Technology 37: 79

Goldstein D J, Horobin R W 1974 Rate factors in staining by Alcian Blue. Histochemical Journal 6: 157

Gomori G 1946 A new histochemical test for glycogen 2nd mucin. American Journal of Clinical Pathology 16: 177

Gomori G 1950 A rapid one-step trichrome stain. American Journal of Clinical Pathology 20: 661

Green F J 1990 The Sigma–Aldrich handbook of stains, dyes and indicators. Aldrich, Milwaukee, WI

Grimelius L 1968 A silver nitrate stain for α_2 cells in human pancreatic islets. Acta Societa Medica Uppsala 73: 243

Grocott R G 1955 A stain for fungi in tissue sections and smears. American Journal of Clinical Pathology 25: 975

Grubic Z, Brzin M 1979 Quantitative evaluation of the trapping reaction of copperthiocholine histochemical procedures for localisation of cholinesterases. Histochemistry 56: 213

Hall M J 1960 A staining reaction for bilirubin in tissue sections. American Journal of Clinical Pathology 34: 313

Hartley F R 1969 The chemistry of chrome mordanting wool. Journal of the Society of Dyers and Colourists 85: 66

Horobin R W 1983 Staining plastic sections: a review of problems, explanations and possible solutions. Journal of Microscopy 131: 173

Horobin R W 1988 Understanding histochemistry: selection, evaluation and design of biological stains. Horwood, Chichester

Horobin R W, Bennion P J 1973 The interrelation of the size and substantivity of dyes: the role of van der Waals attractions and hydrophobic bonding in biological staining. Histochemie 33: 191

Horobin R W, Flemming L 1980 Structure–staining relationships in histochemistry and biological staining. II. Mechanistic and practical aspects of the staining of elastic fibres. Journal of Microscopy 119: 357

Horobin R W, Flemming L 1988 One-bath Trichrome staining – an investigation of a general mechanism, based on a structure-staining correlation analysis. Histochemical Journal 20: 29

Horobin R W, Goldstein D J 1972 Impurities and staining characteristics of Alcian Blue. Histochemical Journal 4: 391

Horobin R W, Goldstein D J 1974 The influence of salt on the staining of tissue sections with basic dyes: an investigation into the general applicability of the critical electrolyte concentration theory. Histochemical Journal 6: 599

Horobin R W, James N T 1970 The staining of elastic fibres with Direct Blue 152. A general hypothesis for the staining of elastic fibres. Histochemie 22: 324

Horobin R W, Murgatroyd L B 1971 The staining of glycogen with Best's carmine and similar hydrogen bonding dyes. A mechanistic study. Histochemical Journal 3: 1

Horobin R W, Walters K 1987 Understanding Romanowsky staining. 1. The Romanowsky–Giemsa effect in blood smears. Histochemistry 86: 331

Horobin R W, Flemming L, Kevill-Davies I M 1974 Basic Fuchsin–ferric chloride: a simplification of Weigert's resorcin–Fuchsin stain for elastic fibres. Stain Technology 49: 207

Horobin R W, Gerrits P O, Wright D 1991 Staining sections of water-miscible resins. 2. Effects of staining-reagent lipophilicity on the staining of glycol-methacrylate-embedded tissues. Journal of Microscopy 166: 199

Hoyer P E, Lyon H, Jakobsen P, Andersen A P 1986 Standardised Methyl Green–pyronin Y procedures using pure dyes. Histochemical Journal 18: 90

Hyman E S 1992 Improved microscopic detection of bacteriuria. Biotechnic and Histochemistry 67: 1

International Committee for Standardization in Haematology 1984 ICSH reference method for staining of blood and marrow films by Azur B and eosin Y (Romanowsky–Giemsa stain). British Journal of Haematology 57: 707

Iwamoto T, Yamashita K, Iijimata S 1979 A spectrophotometric method for selecting Orcein dyes for histological demonstration of hepatitis B surface antigen. Acta Histochemica et Cytochemica 12: 63

James J, Tas J 1984 Histochemical protein staining. Royal Microscopical Society/Oxford University Press, Oxford

Johannes M-L, Klessen C 1984 Alcian blue/PAS or PAS/Alcian blue? Remarks on a classical technic used in carbohydrate histochemistry. Histochemistry 80: 129

References

Jones D B 1957 Nephrotic glomerulonephritis. American Journal of Pathology 33: 313

Kashiwa H K, House C M 1964 The glyoxal bis(2-hydroxyanil) method modified for localised insoluble calcium salts. Stain Technology 39: 359

Kashiwa H K, Park H Z 1976 Light microscopic localisation of labile calcium in hypertrophied chrondrocytes of long bone with Alizarin Red S. Journal of Histochemistry and Cytochemistry 24: 634

Kelenyi G 1967 On the histochemistry of the azo group-free thiazole dyes. Journal of Histochemistry and Cytochemistry 15: 172–180

Kiernan J A 1984a Chromoxane Cyanine T. 1. Physical and chemical properties of the dye and of some of its iron complexes. Journal of Microscopy 134: 13

Kiernan J A 1984b Chromoxane Cyanine T. 2. Staining of animal tissues by the dye and its iron complexes. Journal of Microscopy 134: 25

Kiernan J A 1990 Histological and histochemical methods: theory and practice, 2nd edn. Pergamon, Oxford

Lendrum A C 1947 The phloxine–tartrazine method as a general histological stain and for the demonstration of inclusion bodies. Journal of Pathology and Bacteriology 59: 399

Lendrum A C, Fraser D S, Slidders W, Henderson R 1962 Studies on the character and staining of fibrin. Journal of Clinical Pathology 15: 401

Lillie R D 1977 Conn's biological stains. A handbook on the nature and uses of the dyes employed in the biological laboratory, 9th edn. Williams & Wilkins, Baltimore

Lillie R D, Fulmer H M 1976 Histopathologic technic and practical histochemistry, 4th edn. McGraw-Hill, New York

Lojda Z, Gossrau R, Scheibler T H 1979 Enzyme histochemistry: a laboratory manual. Springer-Verlag, Heidelberg

Lycette R M, Danforth W F, Koppel J L, Olwen J H 1970 The binding of Luxol Fast Blue ARN by various biological lipids. Stain Technology 45: 155

Lyon H 1991 Theory and strategy in histochemistry. A guide to the selection and understanding of techniques. Springer-Verlag, Berlin

Lyon H, Andersen A P, Andersen I, Clausen P P, Herold B 1982 Purity of commercial non-certified European samples of pyronin Y. Histochemical Journal 14: 621

McMullen L, Walker M M, Bain L A, Karim Q N, Baron J H 1987 Histological identification of *Campylobacter* using Gimenez technique in gastric antral mucosa. Journal of Clinical Pathology 40: 464

Magee-Russell S M 1958 Histochemical methods for calcium. Journal of Histochemistry and Cytochemistry 6: 22

Marshall P N 1980 Romanowsky and reticulocyte stains. In: Schmidt R M (ed) CRC handbook series in clinical laboratory science. Section 1: Hematology. CRC Press, Boca Raton, FL, vol 2, p 63

Marshall P N, Horobin R W 1972 The oxidation products of haematoxylin and their role in biological staining. Histochemical Journal 4: 493

Marshall P N, Horobin R W 1973 The influence of inorganic salts when staining with preformed metal complex dyes. Histochemie 37: 299

Marshall P N, Horobin R W 1974a A simple assay procedure for carmine and carminic acid samples. Stain Technology 49: 19

Marshall P N, Horobin R W 1974b A simple assay procedure for mixtures of hematoxylin and hematein. Stain Technology 39: 137

Marshall P N, Bentley S A, Lewis S M 1975 A standardized Romanowsky stain prepared from purified dyes. Journal of Clinical Pathology 28: 920

Marshall P N, Galbraith W, Baccus J W 1979 Studies on Papanicolaou staining. 2. Quantitation of dye components bound to cervical cells. Analytical Quantitative Cytology 1: 169

Meloan S N, Valentine L S, Puchtler H 1971 On the structure of carminic acid and Carmine. Histochemie 27: 87

Miller P J 1971 An elastin stain. Medical Laboratory Technology 28: 148

Mittwer T, Bartholamew J W, Kallman B J 1950 The mechanism of the Gram reaction. 2. The function of iodine in the Gram stain. Stain Technology 25: 169

Mowry R W, Scott J E 1967 Observations of the basophilia of amyloid. Histochemie 10: 8–32

Mowry R W, Longley J B, Emmel V M 1980 Only aldehyde fuchsin made from pararosanilin stains pancreatic beta cell granules and elastic fibres in unoxidised microsections: problems caused by mislabelling of certain basic fuchsins. Stain Technology 55: 91

Nachlas M M, Crawford D T, Seligman A M 1957 Histochemical demonstration of leucine aminopeptidase. Journal of Histochemistry and Cytochemistry 5: 264

Nettleton G S, Carpenter A-M 1977 Studies of the mechanism of the periodic acid–Schiff histochemical reaction for glycogen using infrared spectroscopy and model compounds. Stain Technology 52: 63

Pearse A G E, Stoward P J 1991 Histochemistry, theoretical and applied, vol 3, 4th edn. Churchill Livingstone, Edinburgh

References

Perls M 1967 Nachweis von Eisenoxyd in geweissen Pigmentation. Virchow's Archive für Pathologische Anatomie und Physiologie und für Klinische Medizin 39: 42

Peters A 1955a Experiments on the mechanism of silver staining. 1. Impregnation. Quarterly Journal of Microscopical Science 96: 84

Peters A 1955b Experiments on the mechanism of silver staining. 2. Development. Quarterly Journal of Microscopical Science 96: 103

Popescu A, Doyle R J 1996 The Gram stain after more than a century. Biotechnic and Histochemistry 71: 145

Prento P 1993 Van Gieson's picrofuchsin. The staining mechanisms for collagen and cytoplasm, and an examination of the dye diffusion rate model of differential staining. Histochemistry 99: 163

Proctor G B, Horobin R W 1983 The aging of Gomori's Aldehyde fuchsin: the nature of the chemical changes and the chemical structures of the coloured components. Histochemistry 77: 255

Proctor G B, Horobin R W 1988 Chemical structures and staining of Weigert's resorcin–Fuchsin and related elastic fibre stains. Stain Technology 63: 101

Puchtler H, Sweat Waldrop F 1978 Silver impregnation methods for reticulum fibres and reticulin: a re-investigation of their origins and specificity. Histochemistry 57: 177

Puchtler H, Meloan S N, Terry M S 1969 On the history and mechanism of alizarin and alizarin red S stains for calcium. Journal of Histochemistry and Cytochemistry 17: 110

Puchtler H, Sweat Waldrop F, Meloan S N 1980 On the mechanism of Mallory's phosphotungstic acid–haematoxylin stain. Journal of Microscopy 119: 383

Puchtler H, Sweat Waldrop F, Meloan S N 1983 Application of thiazole dyes to amyloid under conditions of direction cotton dyeing: correlation of histochemical and chemical data. Histochemistry 77: 431–445

Robins J H, Abrams G D, Pincock J A 1980 The structure of Schiff reagent aldehyde adducts and the mechanism of the Schiff reaction as determined by nuclear magnetic resonance spectroscopy. Canadian Journal of Chemistry 58: 330

Roozemond R C 1971 The staining and chromium binding of rat brain tissue and of lipids in model systems subjected to Baker's acid hematein technique. Journal of Histochemistry and Cytochemistry 19: 244

Salthouse T N 1962 Luxol Fast Blue ARN: a new solvent azo dye with improved staining qualities for myelin and phospholipids. Stain Technology 37: 313

Sawyer D, Sie H-G, Fishman W H 1965 A technique for preparing permanent histochemical preparations of liver phosphorylase. Journal of Histochemistry and Cytochemistry 13: 605

Scherrer R 1984 Gram's staining reaction, Gram's types and cell walls of bacteria. Trends in Biochemical Sciences 9: 242

Schulte E, Wittekind D 1989 Standardization of the Feulgen–Schiff technique. Staining characteristics of pure fuchsin dyes: a cytophotometric method. Histochemistry 91: 321

Scott J E 1973 Affinity, competitive and specific interactions in the biochemistry and histochemistry of polyelectrolytes. Transactions of the Biochemical Society 1: 787

Scott J E, Dorling J 1969 Periodic oxidation of acid polysaccharides. 3. A PAS method for chondroitin sulphates and other glycosaminoglycans. Histochemie 19: 295

Scott J E, Mowry R W 1970 Alcian Blue – a consumers' guide. Journal of Histochemistry and Cytochemistry 18: 842

Seidler E 1991 The tetrazolium–formazan system: design and histochemistry. Fischer, Stuttgart

Shikata T, Uzawa T, Yoshiwara N, Akatsuka T, Yamazaki S 1974 Staining methods for Australian antigen in paraffin section-detection of cytoplasmic inclusion bodies. Japanese Journal of Experimental Medicine 44: 25

Shoobridge M P K 1983 A new principle in polychrome staining: a system of automated staining, complementary to hematoxylin and eosin, and usable as a research tool. Stain Technology 58: 245

Shum M W K, Hon J K Y 1969 A modified phosphotungstic acid haematoxylin stain for formalin fixed tissues. Journal of Medical Laboratory Technology 26: 38

Stevens A, Wilson I 1996 The haematoxylins and eosin. In: Bancroft J D, Stevens A (eds) Theory and practice of histological techniques, 4th edn. Churchill Livingstone, New York, p 112

Tas J 1977 The Alcian Blue and combined Alcian Blue–Safranin O staining of glycosaminoglycans studied in a model system and in mast cells. Histochemical Journal 9: 205

Teichman J S, Krick T P, Nettleton G S 1980 Effects of different fuchsin homologues on the Feulgen reagent. Journal of Histochemistry and Cytochemistry 28: 1062

Terner J Y 1966 Phosphotungstic acid–hematoxylin. Reactivity in vitro. Journal of Histochemistry and Cytochemistry 14: 345

Terner J Y, Gurland J, Gaer F 1964 Phosphotungstic acid–hematoxylin; spectrophotometry of the lake in solution and in stained tissue. Stain Technology 39: 141

Trip E J, Mackay E H 1972 Silver staining of bone prior to

decalcification for quantitative determination of osteoid in sections. Stain Technology 47: 129

Tsutsumi Y, Onada N, Osamura R Y 1990 Victoria Blue–Hematoxylin and Eosin staining a useful routine stain for demonstration of invasion by cancer cells. Journal of Histotechnology 13: 271

Tucker F L, Bartholamew J W 1962 Variations in the Gram staining results caused by air moisture. Stain Technology 37: 157

Tunnell G L, Hart M N 1977 Simultaneous determination of skeletal muscle fibre types I, IIA, and IIB by histochemistry. Archive of Neurology 34: 171

Uzman L L 1956 Histochemical localisation of copper with rubeanic acid. Laboratory Investigations 5: 299

Vassar P S, Culling F A 1959 Fluorescent stains with special reference to amyloid and connective tissue. Archives of Pathology 68: 487–498

Von Kossa J 1901 Nachweis von Kalk. Beitrage zur pathologischen Anatomie und zur allegemeinen Pathologie 29: 163

Warthin A S, Starry A C 1920 A more rapid and improved method of demonstrating spirochaetes in tissues. American Journal of Syphilis, Gonorrhea and Venereal Diseases 4: 97

Wittekind D H 1986 On the nature of the Romanowsky–Giemsa staining and the Romanowsky–Giemsa efffect. In: Boon M E, Kok L P (eds) Standardisation and quantitation of diagnostic staining in cytology. Coulomb Press, Leiden, p 27

Wittekind D H, Gehring T 1985 On the nature of the Romanowsky–Giemsa effect. 1. Model experiments on the specificity of Azur B–eosin Y stain as compared with other thiazine dye–eosin Y combinations. Histochemical Journal 17: 263

Wittekind D H, Schulte E, Schmidt G, Frank G 1991 The standard Romanowsky–Giemsa stain in histology. Biotechnic and Histochemistry 66: 283

Where to find technical details of staining methods

▶ General comments

When the necessary critical studies have been carried out, a 'standard' method is cited. However, this is uncommon. Moreover, for many methods there is no single procedure, whether standardized or not, acceptable to all experienced users; hematoxylin and Eosin, Papanicolaou and Romanowsky stains are cases in point. Each variant, with its particular advantages and disadvantages and its particular color balance, is espoused by skilled users. Consequently, the reader is sometimes referred to accounts offering general discussion of a method, rather than a simple entry. For the reader's convenience the following brief listing often refers to a single, wide-circulation, staining manual. There are many other excellent texts, and their omission in no way constitutes criticism of them.

Acid hematin See Bancroft & Stevens (1996: 228) under the rubric 'Dichromate acid hematein (DAH) method' for a typical procedure of this type.

Acid phosphatase, azodye procedure See Bancroft & Stevens (1996: 398) for a typical method.

Adenosine triphosphatase (ATPase), calcium–cobalt method for fiber typing See Bancroft & Stevens (1996: 413) for a routine procedure.

Alcian Blue, critical electrolyte procedure See Bancroft & Stevens (1996: 191) under the rubric 'Alcian blue technique involving critical electrolyte concentration'; see also the proceeding pages for related methods.

Alcian Blue/PAS See Bancroft & Stevens (1996: 192) under the rubric 'Combined Alcian Blue–PAS technique'; see also the following and earlier pages for related methods.

Aldehyde Fuchsin There is no standard procedure; a typical variant is given by Bancroft & Stevens (1996: 134).

Alizarin Red for calcium There is no single standard procedure; a typical variant is given by Bancroft & Stevens (1996: 258).

Alkaline phosphatase, azodye methods See Bancroft & Stevens (1996: 396) for a routine procedure.

Best's Carmine for glycogen See Bancroft & Stevens (1996: 186).

Chloroacetate esterase, for mast and myeloid cells See Bancroft & Stevens (1996: 416) for a routine procedure.

Chromoxane Cyanine for myelin See *Solochrome Cyanine for myelin*, below.

Cresyl Fast Violet for nervous tissue There is no single standard procedure; a typical variant is given by Bancroft & Stevens (1996: 343) under the rubric 'Cresyl Fast Violet (Nissl) stain'.

Fast Green for basic proteins See Chayen & Bitensky (1991: 63).

Feulgen stain for DNA There is no single standard procedure; a typical variant is that given by Bancroft & Stevens (1996: 145); see also immediately prior text.

Gimenez method for *Helicobacter pylori* See Bancroft & Stevens (1996: 297).

Gordon & Sweet's stain for reticulin See Bancroft & Stevens (1996: 135) and immediately prior text.

Gram stain and variants for bacteria There are many variants, for a selection of which see Bancroft & Stevens (1996: 294). For a largely ignored, standardized procedure, see Bartholamew (1962).

Grimelius' silver method for argyrophil cells See Bancroft & Stevens (1996: 285).

Grocott hexamine silver for fungi For two typical variants, see Bancroft & Stevens (1996: 301, 525).

Hematoxylin and Eosin as an oversight stain There are many variants, each used in many laboratories. For a general account of the more widely used methods, see Bancroft & Stevens (1996: ch 6).

Jones's hexamine silver method for basement membranes This is described in Bancroft & Cook (1994: 63).

Lactase, indigogenic method See Bancroft & Stevens (1996: 419).

Leucine aminopeptidase A routine method is given by Bancroft & Stevens (1996: 405).

Luxol Fast Blue for myelin A typical variant is given by Bancroft & Stevens (1996: 353).

Masson–Fontana procedure for melanin Over the years many variants have been described. A typical method is given by Bancroft & Stevens (1996: 252).

Masson's Trichrome There is no single standard procedure. A typical variant is that given by Bancroft & Stevens (1996: 129); see also immediately prior text.

Methyl Green–pyronin for plasma cells There are many variant methods. However, there is a standardized procedure using commercially available pure dyes (Hoyer et al 1986).

Miller's elastin stain See Bancroft & Cook (1994: 56).

Modified Ziehl–Neelsen procedure for leprosy bacilli A typical method of this sort is described in Bancroft & Stevens (1996: 298) under the heading 'Wade–Fite technique for leprosy bacilli'.

MSB technique for fibrin and other acidophilic materials For the sequence stain variant, see Bancroft & Stevens (1996: 130); for the one-bath stain, see Bancroft & Cook (1994: 76).

Myoadenylate deaminase The method given in Bancroft & Stevens (1996: 415) is essentially that first suggested for diagnosis.

NADH diaphorase See Bancroft & Stevens (1996: 409) for the routine method.

Nile Blue for lipids See Bancroft & Stevens (1996: 221) under the rubric 'Nile Blue sulphate method'.

Nonspecific esterase, the α-naphthyl acetate method See Bancroft & Stevens (1996: 402) for a typical procedure.

Oil Red O for fats For a routine method, see Bancroft & Stevens (1996: 220).

Papanicolaou stains There are many variants, each used by many laboratories. For a typical procedure, see Bancroft & Stevens (1996: 523). For a general account, considering many variants and offering extensive background discussion, see Boon & Druijver

(1986); in particular, see chapter 6, and also the index entry 'Papanicolaou'.

PAS for polysaccharides There is no single standard procedure; a typical variant is given by Bancroft & Stevens (1996: 185); see also immediately prior text.

Perls' Prussian blue for ferric iron See Bancroft & Stevens (1996: 245).

Phloxine–tartrazine technique for viral inclusions See Bancroft and Stevens (1996: 304).

Phosphorylase See Bancroft & Stevens (1996: 414) for a routine procedure.

Phosphotungstic acid–hematoxylin Several variants of this stain are described in Bancroft & Stevens (1996: 107, 357).

Romanowsky–Giemsa stains There are many variant methods. However, standardized procedures using commercially available pure dyes are available. See Marshall et al (1975), and also the method recommended by the International Committee for Standardization in Haematology (1984).

Shikata Orcein for hepatitis B antigen See Bancroft & Stevens (1996: 304).

Solochrome Cyanine for myelin See Bancroft & Stevens (1996: 353) for a typical procedure, and Kiernan (1984b) for the most de-mythologized practical account available.

Southgate's Mucicarmine for mucins See Bancroft & Stevens (1996: 197).

Sucrase, by an azodye method See Bancroft & Stevens (1996: 419) for the routine method.

Sudan Black for lipids See Bancroft & Stevens (1996: 220) for a discussion of various methods of this type.

Thiocholine cholinesterase method See Bancroft & Stevens (1996: 404) for a routine method.

Thioflavine T methods for amyloid The original Vassar and Culling method, and the Burns modification, may both be found in Bancroft & Stevens (1996: 196).

Toluidine Blue for basophilia and metachromasia There is no single standard procedure. A typical variant is given by Bancroft & Stevens (1996: 163).

Van Gieson's and other picrotrichrome oversight and collagen

Where to find technical details of staining methods

stains There is no single standard procedure. A typical variant is given by Bancroft & Stevens (1996: 127).

Von Kossa method for mineralized bone There are several variants of this procedure, a typical one being that given by Bancroft & Stevens (1996: 332). The block-impregnation procedure is described by Bancroft & Cook (1994: 408).

Warthin–Starry method for spirochetes This is described in Bancroft & Stevens (1996: 298).

Ziehl–Neelsen and related stains of acid-fast bacteria A selection of the many variants of this procedure may be found in Bancroft & Stevens (1996: 256, 295–296).

Index

Numbers in **bold** type refer to color plates.

Acetylcholinesterase, 210
Acid hematin for phospholipids, 2–5
Acid mucins *see* Mucins
Acid phosphatase
   azodye methods, **4**, 26–30
   review, 30
Acid-fast bacteria, **35**, 236–240
Acidophilic materials, 128–131
Adenosine triphosphate (ATPase) demonstration
   fiber typing, **3**, 22–24
   impurity problems, 23
   review, 24
Alcian Blue
   acid mucins, 6
   critical electrolyte concentration (CEC) method, 6–9
   impurity problems, 7–8
   nomenclature, 6
Alcian Blue-periodic acid-Schiff (PAS) method, mucins, **1**, 10–13
Aldehyde Fuchsin, 14–17
   B cells, **2**
   elastic fibers, **2**, 14
   Gabe's, 16
   impurity problems, 16–17
   pancreatic beta-cell granules, 14
   review, 17
Alizarin Red S, 18–21
   impurity problems, 21
Alkaline phosphatase
   azodye methods, 32–35
   review, 35

Amyloid
   Congo Red (Highman's method), **6**, 44–47
   Thioflavine T method, 214–216
Anionic glycosaminoglycans, 6, 10
Argentaffin, **16**, 110–112
Arginine-rich proteins, 52
Argyrophil cells, **12**, 82–83
Aschoff-Rokitansky sinuses, 63
Azodye methods
   acid phosphatase, **4**, 26–30
   alkaline phosphatase, 32–35
   nonspecific esterase, **20**, 138–140
   Succinate dehydrogenase, **31**, 198–200
   Sucrase, 202–204

Baker's acid hematin, 3
Baker's Mucicarmine, 195
Basal laminae, 94–96
Basement membranes, **14**, 94–96
Basic proteins, 52–54
Basophilia, **32**, 218–221
Best's Carmine
   alternative dyes, 36–37
   glycogen, 36–39
Bile pigments, **8**, 62–63
Biological Stain Commission, 78
Blood, 176
Bone
   Alizarin Red, 18
   Von Kossa, 228
Bridges and Luna method, 233
Burn's variant, 214

Calcium, 229
   Alizarin Red S, 18–21

263

Index

Carmine, impurity problems, 195
Carminic acid, 36
Cartilage matrix staining, 11
Carzzi's hematoxylin, 89
Chitin, 86
Chloroacetate esterase demonstration
   myeloid and mast cells, **5**, 40–44
   review, 43
Cholesterol, 206
Cholinesterases, 138, 210
Chromatin, 118
Chromosomal bands, 176
Chromoxane Cyanine R, 191
Chymotrypsin-like proteases, 40
Cole's hematoxylin, 89
Collagen stains, 222–226
Color Index (CI) nomenclature, xiii
Congo Red for amyloid (Highman's method), **6**, 44–47
Copper associated protein (CAP), 182
Copper, Rubeanic acid, 182–184
Cresyl Fast Violet, nucleic acids, 48–50
Cresyl Violet, 48
Cytogenetics, 176–181
Cytological preparations, 176
Cytology, Papanicolaou stains, **22**, 150–153

Delafield's hematoxylin, 89
Dichromate-acid hematin, 3
Dithiooxamide, 182
DNA
   Feulgen stain, **7**, 56–61
   Methyl Green, 118
Dyes
   Alcian Blue, 6
   Luxol Fast Blue, 106
   impurities of
      Alcian Blue, 7, 9
      Aldehyde Fuchsin, 15–17
      Carmine, 195–196
      Orcein, 187
      Pyronin, 122
      Romanowsky-Giemsa stains, 178–180
      Tetrazolium salts, 199–200
   nomenclature, xii
   Solochrome Cyamine, 190

Ehrlich's hematoxylin, 89
Elastic fibers, 14
   Aldehyde Fuchsin, 14
   Miller's stain, **18**, 124–126
   Victoria Blue, 126

Esterase demonstration, 138
   review, 140, 212

Fast Green FCF
   basic proteins, 52–54
   review, 54
Fat, Oil Red O, 146
Fatty acids, 206
Faulkner and Lillie method, 233
Ferric iron, **24**, 160–163
Feulgen stain
   DNA, **7**, 56–61
   review, 60–61
   standardized staining method, 61
Fiber typing
   ATPase demonstration, **3**, 22–24
   Myoadenylate deaminase, 132
   NADH diaphorase, 134
   Phosphorylase demonstration, **26**, 168–170
Fibrin, MSB technique, 128–131
Fite method, 243
Fouchet technique, **8**, 62–63
Fungi, **13**, 84–87

Gabe's Aldehyde Fuchsin, 16
Giemsa's stain, 178
Gimenez method, 64–66
Glycogen, 86
   Best's Carmine, 36–39
Glycoproteins, 10
Gmelin technique, 63
Goblet cells, 11
Gomori's one-step trichrome, **9**, 68–70
Gomori's silver stain, 73, 95
Gordon and Sweet's silver stain, 95
   reticulin, **10**, 72–75
Gram stain
   bacteria, **11**, 76–81
   review, 81
   standardized staining method, 81, 258
Gram-Twort stain, 76–81
Grimelius' silver method, **12**, 82–83
Grocott hexamine (methamine) silver, **13**, 84–87

Helicobacter pylori, 64–66
Hematoxylin and Eosin
   oversight stain, 88–93
Hemoglobin, 160
Hemorrhagic areas, 63
Hemosiderin, 160

Index

Hepatitis B antigen, **30**, 186–188
Hexamine silver stain, 84, 94
Hexazotized Pararosanilin, 26–30
  impurity problems, 28
Highman's method, **6**, 44–47

Indigogenic method, 98–99
Infarcted areas, 63
Iron, 160–163

Jones's hexamine silver
  basal laminae, 94–96
  basement membranes, **14**, 94–96

Lactase, indigogenic method, 98–99
Lecithin, 206
Leishman's stain, 178
Leprosy bacilli, **36**, 242–245
Leucine aminopeptidase demonstration, **15**, 100–104
  review, 104
Lipases, 138
Lipids
  background staining, 29
  Nile Blue, 142–145
  Oil Red O, **21**, 146–148
  Sudan Black, 206–209
Liver bile pigment, 62
Luxol Fast Blue, 106–109
Lysine-rich proteins, 52

Marris' hematoxylin, 89
Masson's Trichrome, 114–117
Masson-Fontana method, **16**, 110–112
Mast cells, 40–43
Mayer's hematoxylin, 89
Mayer's Mucicarmine, 195
Melanin, **16**, 110–112
Metachromasia, **32**, 218–221
Methamine silver stain, 84
Methyl Green, 118
Methyl Green-Pyronin
  impurity problems, 122
  plasma cells, **17**, 118–122
  review, 122
  standardized staining method, 119, 259
Microorganisms, 176
Microtomy, problems with, xiv
Miller's elastin stain, **18**, 124–126
Mineralized bone, 18, **33**, 228–230

Modified Ziehl-Neelsen technique, **36**, 242–245
MSB technique
  acidophilic materials, 128–131
  fibrin, **19**, 128
Mucins, 86
  Alcian Blue, 6
  Alcian Blue periodic acid-Schiff (PAS) method, **1**, 10–13
  anionic glycosaminoglycans, 6,10
  glycoproteins, 10
  goblet cells, 11
  Southgate's Mucicarmine stain, 194–197
Muscle biopsies, 134–136
  see also Fiber typing
Mycobacteria, 237
Myelin
  Luxol Fast Blue, 106–109
  Solochrome Cyanine stain, 190–193
Myeloid cell lines, 40–43
Myoadenylate deaminase, 132–133
Myoglobin, 160

NADH diaphorase, 134–136
  review, 136
Nervous tissue, 48–50
Neutral mucins *see* Mucins
Nile Blue
  impurity problems, 144
  lipids, 142–145
  review, 145
Nissl substance, 48
Nomenclature, xii–xiii
Nonspecific esterase, azodye method, **20**, 138–140
Nucleal staining procedure, 56
Nucleic acids, 48–50

Oil Red O
  fats, **21**,146–148
  review, 148
Orcein, 186–188
Osteoid, 228
Oversight staining, 222–226
  Hematoxylin and Eosin, 88–93
  Masson's Trichrome, 114–117
  Phosphotungstic acid hematoxylin, **27**, 172–175
  Toluidine Blue, 218–221

Pancreatic beta-cells, 14

Index

Papanicolaou stains
  cytology, **22**, 150–153
  review, 153
  standardized staining method, 153
Periodic acid-Schiff (PAS) procedure
  mucins, 10–13
  polysaccharides, **23**, 154–158
  review, 158
Perl's Prussian Blue, **24**, 160–163
Phloxine-Tartrazine technique, **25**, 164–166
Phospholipids, 208
  acid hematin, 2–5
  unmasking, 3
Phosphorylase demonstration
  muscle fiber typing, **26**, 168–170
  review, 170
Phosphotungstic acid hematoxylin (PTAH), **27**, 172–175
  impurity problems, 174
Picro-Sirius Red, 224
Picrotrichrome stains, 222–226
Plasma cells, **17**, 118–122
Polysaccharides, **23**, 154–158
Proteases, Leucine aminopeptidase demonstration, **15**, 100–104

Reticulin, **10**, 72–75
Ribosomes, 118
RNA, 118
Romanowsky-Giemsa stains, **28**, 176–181
  review, 180–181
  standardized staining methods, 181, 259
Rubeanic acid, **29**, 182–184

Schiff reagent
  dry, 58
  impurity problems, 58–59, 156
Sections *see* Tissue sections
Shikata Orcein method, **30**, 186–188
Silver methenamine, 85
Skeletal muscle
  ATPase, **3**, 22–24
  MSB technique, 128–131
  Myoadenylate deaminase, 132–133
  NADH diaphorase, 134–136
  phosphorylase demonstration, **26**, 168–170
Solochrome Cyanine R, 190
Solochrome Cyanine stain, 190–193
Southgate's Mucicarmine stain
  mucins, 194–197
  review, 196–197
Spirochetes, **34**, 232–234

Stains, nomenclature, xii–xiii
Starch, 86
Stein technique, 63
Succinate dehydrogenase demonstration
  azodye method, **31**, 198–200
  review, 200
Sucrase, azodye method, 202–204
Sudan Black
  impurity problems, 208
  lipids, 206–209
  review, 209

Thiocholine cholinesterase method, 210–212
Thioflavine T method, 214–216
  review, 216
Tissue sections
  artefacts, xiv–xv
  contamination, xv
  creases, xiv
  dust, xv
  folds, xiv
  hairline cracks, xiv
  hairs, xv
  score marks, xiv
  scratches, xiv
  squames, xv
  thick in neuroanatomical investigations, 48
Toluidine Blue
  basophilia, **32**, 218–221
  metachromasia, **32**, 218–221
  oversight stain, 218–221
Trichromes
  Gomori's, **7**, 68–70
  Masson's, 114–117
  review, 70, 117
  Van Gieson's, 222–226

Van Gieson's stain, 222–226
  review, 226
Victoria Blue, 126
Viral inclusions, **25**, 164–166
Von Kossa technique, **33**, 228–230

Warthin-Starry method, **34**, 232–234
Weigert technique, modified, 124–126
Wilder's silver stain, 73, 95
Wright's stain, 178

Ziehl-Neelsen method
  acid-fast bacteria, **35**, 236–240
    modified for leprosy bacilli, **36**, 242–245